literal interpretation of organized myth. The Scientific Revolution decentered those myths. So is humanity now left without a source of deep meaning and moral compass? Perhaps not. The Mindfulness Revolution offers a totally new direction: industrial-strength psycho-spiritual growth based on industrial-strength attentional skills — concentration power, sensory clarity, and equanimity. This book offers a rich banquet, inviting you to taste many flavors of mindfulness."

— Shinzen Young, director of Vipassana Support International

"*Secular Meditation* is a wonderfully practical book grounded in the latest neuroscience. Rick Heller shows readers how one can mindfully learn to love others and be loved by others. It provides a step-by-step guide for anyone who wants to live a happy life."

— Paul J. Zak, PhD, author of *The Moral Molecule*

"*Secular Meditation* by Rick Heller is a wonderful door-opener for people who are interested in the benefits and how-to of meditation and mindfulness practices but who are skeptical about the religious sources. Heller, the meditation teacher for the Humanist Community at Harvard, has collected thirty-two practices that will have something for every curious reader. His style is warm and engaging, with great stories sprinkled in, and he pulls the reader into trying out attention and kindness practices from all different angles to find their right fit."

— Christiane Wolf, MD, PhD, coauthor of
A Clinician's Guide to Teaching Mindfulness

"In simple, accessible language, *Secular Meditation* introduces practices that profoundly transform our hearts and consciousness. Through a rich weave of stories, teachings, meditations, and inquiry, this book offers trustworthy guidance on the journey of awakening."

— Tara Brach, PhD, author of *Radical Acceptance* and *True Refuge*

D0062138

Secular
Meditation

A Guide from the
Humanist Community at Harvard

Secular
Meditation

32 PRACTICES FOR
CULTIVATING INNER PEACE,
COMPASSION, AND JOY

RICK HELLER

Foreword by Greg Epstein

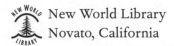 New World Library
Novato, California

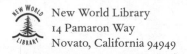

New World Library
14 Pamaron Way
Novato, California 94949

Portions of this book previously appeared in magazine articles in *Buddhadharma*, *Faith Street*, *The Humanist*, *The New Humanism*, *Tikkun*, *UUWorld*, and *Wise Brain Bulletin*.

Text design by Tona Pearce Myers

Library of Congress Cataloging-in-Publication Data
Heller, Rick, date.
Secular meditation : 32 practices for cultivating inner peace, compassion, and joy : a guide from the humanist community at Harvard / Rick Heller ; foreword by Greg Epstein.
    pages   cm
Includes bibliographical references and index.
ISBN 978-1-60868-369-7 (paperback) — ISBN 978-1-60868-370-3 (ebook)
 1. Meditation—Psychological aspects. 2. Happiness. 3. Relaxation. 4. Secularism—21st century. I. Title.
BF637.M4H45 2015
158.1'2—dc23   2015027201

First printing, November 2015
ISBN 978-1-60868-369-7
Printed in Canada on 100% postconsumer-waste recycled paper

New World Library is proud to be a Gold Certified Environmentally Responsible Publisher. Publisher certification awarded by Green Press Initiative. www.greenpressinitiative.org

10   9   8   7   6   5   4   3   2   1

For Cindy

Contents

Part Four: Additional Practices

Foreword

THE DIFFERENCE BETWEEN just being nonreligious and being a humanist in community may come down to practice. At the Humanist Community at Harvard, we've spent the past several years creating a community of nonreligious people, of different backgrounds, who are drawn together by positive humanistic ideals such as reason and compassion. Even though we do not believe in the supernatural, there are positive aspects of participation in a religious community that we too would like to enjoy.

Our community offers lectures, discussion groups, classes for kids, and more. A mainstay of the community is a weekly meeting of a mindfulness and meditation group. Although the group's practices are chiefly adapted from Buddhism, we exclude any beliefs and practices — such as the concept of rebirth — that conflict with mainstream academic science. We see the Buddha as an important cultural, literary, and historic symbol and figure but one who is no more authoritative than Socrates or Benjamin Franklin.

Buddhism appeals to a large number of Westerners who identify as nonreligious. This popularity began in the early twentieth century, when Asian Buddhist leaders such as D. T. Suzuki began traveling to the United States and very purposefully packaged

Buddhist practices to appeal to secularized Westerners looking for answers to questions about life's meaning. A century or so later, with more scientific knowledge and a more diverse and interconnected population, we are seeing an increase in the demand for practices and techniques that can address our spiritual longings without dogma or rigidity.

Perhaps both the greatest promise and the greatest challenge of Buddhism is that it is so diverse. Many people I speak with think that all Buddhism is secular and that it involves no god or gods. However, one of the most widely practiced versions of Buddhism worldwide today is Pure Land Buddhism, which involves prayers meant to transport us in the afterlife to magical heavenly realms where we may encounter giant godlike creatures, hungry ghosts, and other apparitions. These ideas, embraced by many millions of people, don't get much publicity in the West. Neither does the fact that Tibetan Buddhism involves many beliefs, practices, and magical concepts that Westerners would consider irrational, at best, if we even understood or were aware of them.

Tibetan Buddhism has become quite popular in the United States and elsewhere in large part due to the inspirational leadership of the Dalai Lama in response to Tibet's struggle for political autonomy from China. In his approach to Buddhism, the Dalai Lama has gone well beyond even what secular Westerners might think of as reformism. His book *Beyond Religion* indicates a broad skepticism about the existence of anything beyond this natural world — up to and including the theological tradition that identified him as its leader and as the rebirth of a great spirit.

Consistent with the Dalai Lama's liberal approach, the word *mindfulness* has become enormously popular in recent years. It is often associated with key insights and techniques from Buddhist traditions and practices, but without the cultural baggage of a 2,500-year-old Asian tradition. The Dalai Lama has said that in sharing these practices, he's not trying to convert people to Buddhism but rather to inspire them to be more humane and compassionate in whatever religion or philosophy they hold dear. We're delighted to take him up on this compelling call. Mindful of the huge history of cultural appropriation, we do not claim that our Buddhist-influenced humanism is in any sense "true" Buddhism. The label is not important. For us, this practice is about learning, as humbly as we can, from human heritage in a sincere effort to live good, grounded, socially and personally constructive lives.

Today, mindfulness practitioners and teachers include clinical psychiatrists and research psychologists who have sought to distill the essence of Buddhist teachings into a secular form. They also include yogis, spiritual leaders, life coaches, and a huge range of other teachers. If you set out to study Buddhism or mindfulness in the West today, you'll find an enormous variety of options. How to choose?

The Humanist Community at Harvard has long recognized that there's much of value in Buddhism and mindfulness. We are, however, skeptical of any claim of revealed authority, of the notion that any individual or way of thinking has the definitive answer to how we ought to live. Humanists do not believe in gods, but we do believe in *evidence*. Before adopting contemplative practices or spiritual techniques into our lives, we want to see proof that such things are actually effective. That's why, in addition to presenting secular meditation practices, this book also discusses recent scientific research on mindfulness.

Who is this community, however? We're an unusual organization that has come together to foster community for people who would usually be defined by what they're not — people who are atheists, agnostics, secular, nonreligious. It's not a church. It has no dogma. It has no requirements, judges, priests, or inviolable rites. But it does draw on a long tradition of people thinking together about what the good life can mean. And just as the Dalai Lama is not trying to convert you to Buddhism, we're not trying to convert you to humanism. We are simply presenting for your consideration ideas that we have found useful.

Rick Heller has been pioneering this approach to mindfulness practice in our community for five years, and only now does it feel like the idea we had back then is attaining widespread relevance. When you consider the billion nonreligious people on this planet, it becomes evident that there is a desperate need for practices that can help us center ourselves, connect with our values, and help one another emotionally, practically, and politically.

This book is an initial effort to catalog some of those practices. It's not the final word on the subject: it's *a* guide, not *the* guide, for nonreligious people. It is the product of efforts by a group of people who've simply chosen to meet together regularly to help one another try to get a little better at life. Rick writes invitingly and modestly about how you explore a rich inner life. It's my pleasure to invite you to join us on the journey.

Greg Epstein,
Harvard University Humanist Chaplain

Introduction

A COUPLE OF YEARS AGO, I started noticing flashes of light when I was in a darkened room. My eye doctor said I should visit a specialist right away because it could be a sign of a detached retina, which can lead to blindness.

This was alarming news, but I tried to settle my emotions by being "in the moment." On the drive over to the ophthalmologist, I was able to enjoy the colors of fall foliage rather than focus on the medical problem. When I got to the doctor's office, though, it was harder. For one thing, there was no artwork on the wall — nothing to look at except utilitarian office furniture.

Then the medical assistant called me in. She tried to retrieve my record on the computer. It wouldn't come up. She apologized and said she would have to take notes by hand. She was clearly irritated. I decided to offer her my best wishes by practicing a short loving-kindness meditation. This particular meditation uses certain phrases, and the words I said silently went something like this:

I'd like you to be safe
I'd like you to be healthy

I'd like you to be happy
I'd like you to be at ease in the world

I don't know if it made any difference to her, but it sure made a difference to me. Shifting my attention from my problems to her problems, and feeling kindness toward her, gave me a terrific boost. Later I received good news when the doctor diagnosed my condition as a vitreous detachment that did not jeopardize my eyesight.

Loving-kindness meditation is just one of the meditations I'll be sharing in this book. From a secular viewpoint, this practice works not by sending "vibes" through the atmosphere but by changing our own feelings, and subsequently perhaps our actions, in order to be more caring.

I believe that loving-kindness is a critical element of mindfulness. Lately mindfulness has become popular, even trendy. Mindfulness is often defined as *paying nonjudgmental attention to the present moment*. There's increasing scientific evidence that mindfulness can help people reduce their stress and enjoy life. It's getting press for other presumed benefits, too: it's been touted at the World Economic Forum in Davos as a way to increase corporate profits, and the *New York Times*'s influential *Well* blog reported on a study demonstrating that mindfulness helped students improve their test scores. There's even interest in mindfulness as a way of improving accuracy in rifle shooting.[1]

Although mindfulness originated in Buddhism, the recent growth spurt has come in secularized forms that are gaining popularity in health care, business, and the military. Along with growing interest, though, a growing number of people say that something is being lost in the move to secularize mindfulness. In particular, critics fear that, stripped of its ethical moorings, attention training will just help people do what they already do more efficiently: if they are inclined to exploit or harm others, for instance, then exploiting people with focused attention will lead to greater harm.[2]

To avoid such negative effects, mindfulness must be rooted in love. In the original Buddhist approach, it already is. Mindfulness is about paying attention with a particular attitude. This attitude is frequently described as nonjudgmental, but that doesn't necessarily mean neutral or clinical. In fact, the attitude that goes with mindfulness is often described as being friendly, kind, or even loving. Can you really be nonjudgmental and loving at the same time? Yes, if you love just about everything!

This book focuses on training attention and kindness. The goal is to arrive at a place of *nearly* universal love, kindness, or friendliness to whatever is happening in the present. I maintain that universal love is possible. A person does not have to be born with special traits in order to be compassionate and loving. It is a learnable skill.[3]

This book starts with a loving-kindness meditation, one of the meditations I lead for the Humanist Community at Harvard. Although learning to feel more love toward other people may seem like quite a challenge, it's a fairly easy guided meditation. You don't have to clear your mind of thoughts, so even if you think of yourself as someone who can't meditate, you can do this meditation.

Love comes from within. We often think we need to be among friendly people or excellent circumstances to feel love. But in fact, good circumstances are just a crutch that helps us love. If you visit a natural wonder like the Grand Canyon and you love it, it's not because the Grand Canyon loves you. It doesn't even know you exist. You produce these feelings yourself. Love is generated within the brain. We can train ourselves to turn it on. When you love someone or something, even if it doesn't love you back, you still feel good because *you* are feeling love.

Training yourself to love your enemy may be going too far if your enemy is someone who might physically harm you. Yet even if it may be unwise to love bad actors, you don't need to *hate* them. When you hate someone, you're not thinking rationally. The proverb "When you seek revenge, dig two graves" is a reminder that when you act out of hatred, you often harm yourself too. Therefore, it's appropriate to employ a measured amount of loving-kindness even with bad actors, to shift your feelings from hate to *neutrality*. This shift allows you to think *rationally* about people who harm others; you can act to prevent them from doing harm without boiling with outrage and becoming part of the problem yourself.

Loving-kindness meditation is just one of the powerful meditations that we have been practicing at the Humanist Community at Harvard, which serves the needs of nonreligious people in the Boston area. Secular humanists are people who do not believe in the supernatural but do believe in helping fellow human beings. Sometimes this helping takes the form of packing meals for low-income people who might otherwise go hungry. Sometimes we help by sharing techniques such as meditation that soothe emotional distress and add zest to our lives.

Our meditation practices are largely adapted from Buddhism, but we have carefully secularized them. We discard any beliefs or practices that involve the supernatural — such as rebirth — and cast a skeptical eye over anything that remains. You could say that we're rummaging through the Buddhist closet for things that fit. In doing so, we are participating in a larger movement sometimes called "secular mindfulness" or even "secular Buddhism." Just as many humanists are taking up meditation, some Buddhists are discarding supernatural beliefs. Coming from different directions, we have arrived in the same place. Even after the supernatural elements have been shaved off, much in Buddhist philosophy remains valid and can enrich humanism.

Sometimes I hear people question the relevance of a secularized Buddhism. People have asked me, "Isn't Buddhism pretty secular anyway?" Not entirely. The one time I attended a Tibetan meditation, the meditation itself was followed by prayers to a goddess. I have attended a few Zen meditations, but I don't care for the robes, incense, or bowing before a statue of the Buddha. Some argue that these Zen practices aren't really religious, but they certainly feel that way to me. Even the fairly secular Insight Meditation Center community, from which I have learned a great deal, gives a benefit of the doubt to Buddhist philosophy that in my view could benefit from more skepticism.

I have been a facilitator of the Humanist Community at Harvard's mindfulness group for the last five years and lead most of the meditations. Unlike Buddhist groups, which have a hierarchical teacher-student structure, ours is a group of peers. Our discussions are free flowing, in contrast to the practice common in Buddhist circles in which students ask questions and the teacher provides answers, without the students addressing each other directly.

In addition to my experience with meditation, I am a freelance journalist who has published articles about the intersection between Buddhism and neuroscience. I have interviewed psychologists, neuroscientists, and Buddhist teachers; material from these interviews is sprinkled throughout this book. In journalism school, I learned an expression meant to instill a deep skepticism about the things sources tell us: "If your mother says she loves you, *check it out*." So whether the source is Buddhist teachings or scientific research, I try to bring a critical eye to the claims that are made.

This book will show you how to meditate and how to practice mindfulness, which you can think of as a way to carry a meditative state with you throughout the day. Mindfulness, as conceived of here, is a feeling of loving-kindness not just toward people but toward everything! As you go from moment to moment throughout your day, you can have real moments of "wow," of awe and wonder at the rich experience of being alive.

That's not to say that every moment will be perfect. But when a bad moment occurs, mindfulness can help you recover more quickly. This ability is called *resilience*. You can note the unwanted outcome, take appropriate action, and return to a state of equanimity. And even amid challenging times, you can have more and more moments that are truly marvelous.

Part 1 of the book focuses on practices that cultivate kindness and compassion. These are the foundation of humanistic values. This is a good place to start for people who have never meditated before, because it doesn't require learning any new skills. If you have ever loved or even liked another person, you have the prerequisites for learning kindness and compassion meditations.

Part 2 focuses on mindfulness practices that bring inner peace by "quieting the mind" through exercises such as breath meditation and body scan meditation. Until I first experienced it, I didn't even understand what it meant to quiet the mind. I was used to a continuous stream of verbal thoughts running through my head, and I didn't know that this constant chatter could be silenced, let alone how to do it. But through meditation, we can achieve a state of inner quiet that both brings peace and provides a heightened awareness of the world around us.

Part 3 focuses on practices that cultivate joy. In our consumer society, marketers tell us that we need more and more possessions in order to be happy. But as long as our basic needs for food, shelter, clothing, and health care have been met, we have all the physical prerequisites our brains and bodies need to make a mental shift in a more joyful direction.

Part 4 contains additional practices and discussions that go beyond the present-centered focus of mindfulness practices. For instance, it includes a daydreaming meditation in which we allow our minds to wander in order to envision new possibilities for our lives.

One of the things I've learned leading a meditation group is that different people respond best to different types of meditation. So if one meditation doesn't quite work for you, try another. Feel free to jump around in the book; you don't have to read all the chapters or do all the exercises in order.

Each part includes meditation and mindfulness practices as well as personal stories and discussion of scientific research on meditation. By meditation, I mean a period of time dedicated to being mindful of a specific focus, such as the breath. By mindfulness practices, I mean doing everyday tasks such as raking leaves or washing the dishes while paying full attention to the sights, sounds, and sensations around you. I also address frequently asked questions, such as whether there's really such a thing as enlightenment. Although I touch on some of the deeper issues that come up, the focus is on practices that the average person can pursue with a reasonable likelihood of success in a modest amount of time.

Now, let's begin.

Questions to Consider

What is your initial attitude toward meditation?

Do you prefer guided or silent meditations?

How aware are you of your emotions?

How do you feel right now?

When do you find it easy to pay attention? When do you find it difficult?

What are your expectations for this book?

PART ONE

Cultivating Love
and Compassion

CHAPTER ONE

Loving-Kindness Meditation

THIS MEDITATION is a loving-kindness or *metta* meditation. *Metta* is a word from the Pali language of ancient India; it can be translated as "loving-kindness" or "friendliness." It's similar to compassion, except that compassion is concern for the suffering of others. You can have *metta* for someone who's in a good place already.

The purpose of *metta* meditation is to cultivate this feeling of kindness and to learn how to bring it out in circumstances where it may not be your first inclination. Once you've learned to cultivate *metta* toward people, you can extend the practice by having goodwill toward anything, include your own troubling thoughts and feelings. Although this may sound difficult, once you learn how, it becomes a very positive way to live.

Let's go ahead with the meditation. Afterward, I'll discuss some of the issues that sometimes come up during the meditation.

Exercise: Loving-Kindness Meditation

Allow 30 minutes for this exercise. Find a chair or cushion to sit on. If you are using a chair, choose one that allows you to sit up straight. A very simple chair without armrests often works best.

11

Make yourself comfortable. Take off your shoes if you wish. Loosen any tight clothing.

Sit up fairly straight, but not rigidly so. Sometimes it helps to imagine that you're a puppet and there's a cord attached to the top of your head, pulling you up — but gently, not rigidly. If you notice tension in the upper back, tilt your head slightly forward.

Close your eyes, or if you prefer, lower your eyelids and soften your gaze. If you're not sure how to soften your gaze, try *hardening* your gaze by staring intently at one spot on the floor. Note the tension in your facial muscles. Now, stop staring. Notice how the facial muscles relax and how your visual field is broader, though perhaps not as sharp. That is softening your gaze, and it can be very helpful in getting into a meditative state.

Take a deep breath or two. Relax.

The Living Benefactor

Now, think of someone who has helped you at some point in your life, someone toward whom you feel real warmth. And for the language below to work, it has to be someone who is alive.

This individual, who is often called the *benefactor*, doesn't have to be a human being. It could be your cat, dog, or other pet. We're looking for a living being who brings you warm feelings.

If you can visualize the individual, all the better. Imagine they are looking at you with warmth.

With this person in mind, I'd like you to recite a few phrases. I'll use the pronoun *you* because it's gender-neutral. But you can substitute *him*, *her*, or the individual's proper name if you prefer.

The *Metta* Phrases

These phrases are adapted from those of Sharon Salzberg, whose 1995 book *Lovingkindness* popularized *metta* practice in the West.[4]

In the traditional phrasing used by Salzberg and others, the phrases start with "May I," "May she," and so on. To some ears, this sounds like asking God or the universe for a favor. In the Humanist Mindfulness Group, we've adapted the phrases so that they don't have this religious overtone. You're expressing a hope or an intention that affects only you. The words don't magically travel through space to affect the other person. They will affect the other person only if you treat the person with added warmth the next time you encounter them.

So, with your benefactor in mind, say to yourself:

I'd like you to be safe
I'd like you to be healthy
I'd like you to be happy
I'd like you to be at ease in the world

Pause between each phrase. Take a breath to let the meaning sink in.

If you can, imagine what it would look like or sound like to feel that that person was safe, healthy, happy, and at ease.

Repeat the phrases, and see if you can bring *enthusiasm* to them.

I'd like you to be safe
I'd like you to be healthy
I'd like you to be happy
I'd like you to be at ease in the world

A Benefactor Who Is No Longer Living

For many people, it may be easier to think of a benefactor who is no longer alive. It could be a grandparent, another older relative, or perhaps a teacher. Our relationships with the living are sometimes complicated by our desires to get something from them or to change them. Since that is not an option with those who are no longer alive, we can perhaps more easily recall their love for us in an uncomplicated manner. But if no such person comes to mind, you can skip to the next section.

Practicing *Metta* toward Those No Longer Living

Some Buddhists discourage remembrance of people who are no longer alive when doing *metta* practice.[5] For instance, one important Buddhist text relates an anecdote in which a monk was having difficulty with the practice. It turned out that, unbeknownst to him, his benefactor, a former teacher, had recently died. When the monk brought to mind a living benefactor, his practice succeeded.[6] Underlying this anecdote seems to be the belief that something is actually transmitted through psychic powers from the person who offers *metta* to the object of the meditation, and that this transmission would fail if the receiver were dead.

As secularists, however, we see *metta* practice as working solely within our own brains. Someone who lives on in our memories can inspire us just as well as someone who is alive. That's why we created special wording for benefactors who are no longer alive.

With a no-longer-living person in mind and using an appropriate pronoun (*you* doesn't work here, so I'll use *her*), say something like:

> I remember her kindness
> I remember her love
> Memories like these can remind me to be kind to those I encounter.

Again, pause between each phrase, and take a breath.
Repeat the phrases, so that they sink in.

The Self

In the traditional loving-kindness practice that I was taught, one starts with the self and then shifts to the benefactor. We've reversed the order, because a lot of modern people feel self-conscious about directing warm feelings toward themselves and may even wonder whether they deserve them. So we warm up with the benefactor before tackling *metta* toward the self.

Loving yourself is easy to satirize, and if you take the practice too far, you're a narcissist. But really, you deserve as much compassion as the next person. If you feel guilty about loving yourself, then just keep in mind that one of the purposes of this step is to generate warm feelings that you can redirect toward others. Practicing kindness toward yourself will help you be kind toward others.

So, with yourself in mind, say:

I'd like to be safe
I'd like to be healthy
I'd like to be happy
I'd like to be at ease in the world

Give yourself some time to let those words sink in. Can you see yourself in your imagination, safe, healthy, happy, and at ease?

Repeat the phrases.

The Neutral Person

After thinking about benefactors and yourself, you are probably feeling a certain amount of emotional warmth. If you can bring to mind someone you really appreciate, you might even get a little choked up. If you are feeling emotional warmth, your brain has actually been releasing hormones to make you feel this way (more about that later).

Now we come to the trick that makes this an effective means of building empathy toward others.

Think about someone you don't think about much — someone toward whom you feel neutral. It could be a checkout clerk who rang you up at the supermarket or the person who served you coffee this morning at Dunkin' Donuts.

With this neutral person in mind, think:

> I'd like you to be safe
> I'd like you to be healthy
> I'd like you to be happy
> I'd like you to be at ease in the world

As before, recite these phrases slowly, pausing for a breath between each one.

Try to visualize the person if you can. Take note of how it feels to think kindly of this person. Was it surprisingly easy? If so, it may be because the hormones generated when you felt *metta* toward yourself and your benefactors have stuck around. Once generated, these hormones last for a few minutes and bias your feelings toward goodwill.

The Difficult Person

Your emotions are building momentum. Thinking of a benefactor generates warm feelings. Thinking about yourself — I hope — allows the warmth to expand. Thinking about a truly neutral person should not diminish these feelings. Now, we come to the most challenging step, but the one that may be the most useful if you can master it.

Think of someone in your life who bugs you, someone who is irritating — but not the worst person in your life. One of the Buddhist teachers I interviewed, InsightLA's Christiane Wolf, said,

"Don't start with the person who hurt you most in your life. That is just setting yourself up for failure." Coworkers often serve well in this role, because they are people we have to spend time with but might not spend time with voluntarily.

With this challenging person in mind, you can say:

I'd like you to be safe
I'd like you to be healthy
I'd like you to be happy
I'd like you to be at ease in the world

As before, repeat the phrases, taking note of how your mind and your body feel as you say them. Take note of any tightening of the muscles, especially around the gut, which may indicate aversion toward the person. If any of this feels too challenging, you can step back and offer some *metta* to yourself.

I find that wishing a person safety is not a problem. People should be safe, even people I don't like. They should be healthy, too. But wishing them happiness — sometimes I have difficulty with that.

But when I get to wishing them to be "at ease in the world," and I put that together with being happy, it occurs to me that they probably aren't completely happy and completely at ease in the world. If they were, they might not be so difficult. So it's not like you lose something by thinking about this person with kindness.

The steps of this *metta* practice are derived from a Buddhist text called the *Visuddhimagga*. It talks about cultivating loving-kindness toward a hostile person so that you reduce your own ill will and shift from antagonism to feeling neutral.[7] It's not that you feel so warm toward them that you want to hang out with them. The goal is to reach equanimity so that they don't push your buttons.

The phrases above might not be appropriate with regard to someone who is deeply harmful — say, a violent criminal who needs to be incarcerated for everyone's safety. But even in such cases, it may be beneficial to neutralize your hostility toward this person so that you can think rationally about them. That seems perfectly consistent with humanism.

Dealing with "Parking Lot Rage"

A couple of years ago, I took two compassion-themed workshops in quick succession. One was taught by Kristin Neff, a research psychologist at the University of Texas, and Christopher Germer, a clinical psychologist. The other was a *metta* workshop taught by Narayan Helen Liebenson of the Cambridge Insight Meditation Center.

A few days after taking these classes, I got into a dispute in the parking lot of a CVS pharmacy in western Massachusetts. It was a Sunday evening, and the parking lot was deserted. There were maybe a hundred spaces and two or three cars in the parking lot. I swung into a space close to the door, being mindful not to park in the handicapped spot. I did my shopping and got into my car.

That's when I heard a whistle. I was confused for a moment. Then an older guy started lecturing me about letting my car door touch the side of his pickup truck. There was indeed a pickup truck now parked right next to my car, in a lot with a sea of empty spaces.

I told him honestly that when I opened my car door, it had not touched the side of his truck. That should have been the end of it, since no harm had been done. But his blood was up. He retorted that I was a lousy driver who had parked over the white line separating the parking spots, thereby impinging on his spot.

It was true: my car was parked about six inches over the line. I pointed out to him, however, that my car had been there first and that in this almost entirely empty lot, he could have parked one spot over rather than right next to my car.

I don't recall exactly how he responded, except that it was unfriendly.

At that point, I replied, "I don't accept your criticism. Bye," and closed the car door.

The last word I heard him say was "Jackass."

I drove off feeling some tightness in my chest but surprisingly happy. I was pleased that I had not been goaded into anger. Yet the phrase "I don't accept your criticism" didn't sound like anything I'd ever said before. It came out of my mouth spontaneously, and I wondered where from. I concluded that it was probably the result of having practiced *metta* toward myself over the past couple of months.

Universal Love

The culminating step in loving-kindness practice is to cultivate a love for all. This sounds like quite a task — even a burden — if you think about the billions of people in the world, not to mention dogs, cats, farm animals, and wildlife. It's a little easier if you think of it as loving life as a whole, rather than each specific living being.

The traditional wording, a blessing for all beings, doesn't work for me, so I do something different. A Buddhist teacher, Chas DiCapua, used a metaphor I liked: we cultivate an expanding circle of kindness. We start with ourselves and our dear ones. Then we expand it to include people who don't bother us. Then we expand it to include people who do bother us. Then we expand the circle wider and wider until there is no circle anymore. We embrace everyone and everything with *metta*.

So now imagine a circle of concern,
a circle of kindness
expanding out from yourself,
to those near you,
to those further away,
wider and wider
until the circle dissolves
and your intention of being kind
embraces all beings and all things.

That's the loving-kindness practice. If you finish the above in less than thirty minutes, spend the rest of the time meditating silently. You can continue to think about *metta*, or you can meditate on the breath or on sound, two practices I introduce later.

Discussion

At the Humanist Community at Harvard, when we get together as a group to meditate, we usually sit in a circle. After the meditation, we go around the room, introduce ourselves, and talk about how the meditation went. We avoid interrupting each other. After everyone has had a chance to speak, we open up the discussion. People may offer gentle suggestions to others on how to develop a meditation practice.

We also invite people to share joys and concerns. This is a chance for us to talk about what is going on in our lives, whether related to meditation or not. The conversation seems to go best when people talk about personal issues rather than events in the news. Personal matters are kept confidential unless the person says otherwise. We also try to bring a spirit of *metta* to this discussion rather than being argumentative. That's not to say that we don't disagree with each other: we do, but nicely. Often, people go out afterward for a bite to eat, and the conversation continues.

During *metta* meditation, I notice that I warm up as I think about a benefactor and then about myself. But the warmth actually continues to build as I contemplate the neutral person. Sometimes, I also feel more warmth toward myself for being able to think kindly of the neutral person.

I do not consider myself to be a naturally warm person. I believe that most people think I'm nice, but not much more than that. My undergraduate degree is in electrical engineering, and my natural degree of warmth is probably typical of what you would expect of an electrical engineer. I am pleased to have learned how to turn on warmth. I'm still an introvert — as many meditators are — and practicing *metta* does not make me the life of the party. But it does make me feel better, and I hope it makes people feel better when I'm with them.

Questions to Consider

Do you feel warm or cold toward the term *loving-kindness*? Why?

Why might someone else have the opposite feeling toward the term?

Do you find meeting people to be a pleasure or a chore — or does it depend on the circumstances?

Do you consider anyone your enemy or nemesis? If there is such a person, what feelings arise in you when you picture them being happy?

What changes did you notice over the course of the meditation? Was there a point when you noticed a warm glow?

Do you think you can recall the feelings you experienced during the meditation the next time you meet the people you thought about?

CHAPTER TWO

Your Daily Dose of *Metta*

ONE OF THE GOALS of traditional Buddhist practice is to lessen the sense of separation or alienation between people. This is a perfectly appropriate goal for humanists as well, and a good one for the times we live in. American society is growing more diverse. Although one can ask people to celebrate their differences, this is definitely easier said than done.

The social scientist Robert Putnam has found that "in ethnically diverse neighborhoods residents of all races tend to 'hunker down'" and have less contact with their neighbors than in homogeneous neighborhoods. Putnam's data show that thriving and diverse neighborhoods, such as Jamaica Plain in Boston, are more the exception than the rule. In general, the more diverse the community, the less likely people are to say they trust their neighbors.[8] Furthermore, young American adults born after 1980 are least likely to say, "Most people can be trusted" and most likely to say, "You can't be too careful in dealing with people." As I discuss later, psychologists find a clear relationship between love and trust. Declining levels of trust, therefore, can be a sign that people may be less willing to help others or to work toward the common good.[9]

A technique that enabled people to overcome distaste for those who are different would be helpful in overcoming distrust. This is precisely what the practice of *metta* can do. Obviously, some prejudice is conscious and willful. People who intend harm toward others are unlikely to participate in loving-kindness meditation. But to the extent that our ill will is unintended and even unconscious, *metta* practice may help. To overcome unintended ill will, we must first be mindful of our thoughts and feelings. Then, rather than berating ourselves for our moments of ill will, we can substitute *metta* for those feelings, both toward people we have judged and toward our less-than-perfect selves.

Evidence That *Metta* Overcomes Bias

Yoona Kang, a doctoral candidate in cognitive psychology at Yale University, used the Implicit Association Test to study people's unconscious attitudes toward the homeless before and after practicing loving-kindness meditation. This test takes advantage of the fact that people react quickly to words that are easily associated (e.g., *young* and *lovely*) but stumble a bit in associating words that don't go together so easily for them (e.g., *elderly* and *lovely*). Kang tested volunteers and found that unconscious bias against the homeless decreased after six weeks of loving-kindness meditation. A comparison group that met to discuss loving-kindness without practicing meditation showed no decrease in unconscious bias.[10] It appears that loving-kindness meditation affects not just thoughts but emotions as well.

Exercise: Your Daily Dose of *Metta*

It may take twenty minutes or more to go through the steps of the formal *metta* meditation. But off the cushion and out in the world, you may want to do it more quickly.

If you have already practiced *metta* meditation, you know you are capable of shifting your feelings. Let's say you encounter a stranger on the street, in the subway, or in a store. And let's say you make a snap negative judgment about them and notice yourself doing it. And let's say this judgment is not justified by any bad behavior on the part of this other person. If you're mindful of this, you can simply say to yourself, "You too," meaning, "You and I are on the same team." See if a simple "You too" can help you get over this sense of separation.

If that doesn't work and there's time, in your mind's eye, picture a benefactor for a second or two. Then consider the person before you once again. This can help shift your feelings from negative to neutral.

There may be other situations in which you feel neutral toward a person but would like to be a little warmer. You can use this practice to shift feelings from neutral to positive. In your mind, give this person one moment of your attention flavored with a little dose of kindness.

In encountering strangers, of course, you should exercise due caution. Also, depending on the community where you live, even if you feel kindly toward a stranger, it may be best not to express it openly, because it may unnerve the person.

When in Boston...

I often feel like smiling at people when I do this practice, or even saying hello. You can always get away with a smile. But saying hello may not always be socially appropriate.

My friend Deborah Finn, concerned that Boston was perceived to be "cold and unwelcoming to outsiders," made the following pledge on a civic website: "I will smile and say 'hello' to strangers I pass on the streets in my neighborhood but only if 50 residents of Boston, Massachusetts, USA will do the same." Ninety-one people signed up.

Pretty innocuous, right? Well, one writer in *Boston* magazine called her out on her project, complaining that she was trying to turn Boston into Minneapolis. With his tongue not very far into his cheek, he wrote:

> Hoping to friendly up the joint, and so stem the tide of flee-ing Volvos, concerned citizen Deborah Finn and local painter Bren Bataclan have launched the Hello Boston and Smile Bos-ton projects, respectively, encouraging locals to grin, unpro-voked, at people they don't know. Wonderful. While we're at it, why don't we level Beacon Hill and erect a Space Needle? Because, say what you will about pipe-wielding crackheads, the threat they pose to our way of life is nothing compared to the one posed by those intent on suppressing our native character. Being rude is as essential a part of Boston's cultural heritage as the bean or the cod.[11]

Discussion

You may observe that this practice helps you to notice whether you are making negative snap judgments about people. This can be so habitual that you don't notice you're doing it unless you are mindful of it.

You may wonder, though, what good is this *metta* practice unless you express it or do something about it? If it's just internal, what good does it do?

First, it will increase your positive emotions. Second, it's likely that people will be more comfortable around you even if you don't say anything. Our feelings are expressed in our body language, so other people do pick up on how we're feeling toward them.

But this does raise the question of whether, if you are culti-vating loving-kindness, you should follow that up with concrete actions that will help people in need. In my opinion, you probably should, at least by paying your fair share of taxes and, if you can, making additional contributions to charity.

The Humanist Community at Harvard has a program called Values in Action. At one such event, we packed meals for food-insecure families. The meal packing is done in an assembly line. I wondered if bringing *metta* to it would enhance the experience, but my effort to visualize the families who would enjoy the meals was not very successful. Practicing *metta* toward the other volunteers on the assembly line was helpful, but overall, I found that bringing mindfulness to my bodily movements was the best way for me to deal with the challenge of the repetitive work.

Becoming Friendlier

Metta can help us bridge the emotional distance we feel toward some people, but it can also make us more outgoing in less threatening circumstances. When I was starting to practice *metta* seriously, I happened to attend a talk by a noted environmentalist. The talk was preceded by a dinner. I didn't have anyone to talk to as I stood in line to get food, so I decided to do *metta* toward the people around me. This opened me up enough that I decided to introduce myself to the man in front of me. Once I started talking to him, I realized he was a Buddhist-influenced environment writer whose blog I read, and we had a nice conversation. It was no great surprise that this person was at this talk, but if I had not warmed up my emotions with *metta* practice, I would never have known it.

CHAPTER THREE

Compassion Meditation

OUR COMPASSION PRACTICE is adapted from a Tibetan Buddhist meditation known as *tonglen*. The practice is to be mindful of suffering while breathing in and to be mindful of love and compassion while breathing out. In one form of the traditional practice, you imagine sending out white light as you breathe out.[12] We've dispensed with that.

As to *whose* suffering to think about, that's up to you. Typically, *tonglen* meditation involves empathy for the suffering of others. There is a lot of suffering in the world, so don't try to take on everyone who suffers; pick one person or a few people. If you feel too overwhelmed by your own issues to contemplate the suffering of others, then you might start with yourself. Another time, when you're more together, you can practice this meditation with others in mind.

The words *compassion* and *empathy* are sometimes mixed up, so much so that even Tania Singer, a scientist who studies the neural signatures of these feelings in the brain, reports miscommunication with her study subjects.[13] *Empathy* means feeling what another person is feeling, so if another person is feeling anger and you empathize with that person, you become angry. When you empathize with the suffering of others, you yourself suffer.

Compassion, in this practice, is a positive emotion. The feeling you cultivate on the out-breath is similar in feeling to the *metta* we practiced earlier. According to the way Buddhists use the terms, one feels compassion toward a being that is suffering. *Metta* is a feeling of kindness that can be directed toward anyone, including people who are not suffering at all. But there may not be much difference in what you feel during these two practices. You are likely to experience the same basic feeling of warmth and connection whether you are extending *metta* or compassion.

This practice is about cultivating feelings. It's not an intellectual exercise aimed at identifying the problem or injustice that is causing the suffering. It's not about fixing that problem. It's about connecting emotionally with people who suffer and comforting them. Thinking about how to solve problems is obviously valuable, but it's not part of this meditative practice.

Exercise: Compassion Meditation

Allow 20 minutes for this exercise. Start by taking a few deep breaths to relax. If you feel you need to warm up to this meditation, you can start with an abbreviated *metta* meditation, perhaps calling to mind the loving-kindness you've received from a benefactor.

Now, as you breathe in, think of someone who is suffering. You may want to visualize the person and notice the expression on their face. Be mindful of the feelings you have as you have empathy for the person and the suffering they are going through.

Then, as you breathe out, imagine you are comforting this person. What does that feel like and look like?

Cycle back and forth between noticing suffering and imagining comfort. Try to time this with the in-breath and the out-breath. But if that becomes a chore, don't worry about synchronizing with the breath.

You don't need to focus on one person the whole time. You can think about a variety of people, remembering their suffering and imagining comforting them. But if you think about more than one person, it will probably work better if you think about them one at a time rather than collectively. Because of the way the brain works, it's easier to feel compassion for individuals than for groups.

You can include yourself among those suffering, if it feels right. And if you start to feel discomfort about the meditation — perhaps because you connect too strongly with another person's suffering — you can focus on that discomfort on the in-breath, and give yourself self-compassion on the out-breath.

Discussion

At the Humanist Community at Harvard, we did a compassion meditation the day after the bombing of the 2013 Boston Marathon, which left three people dead and many more grievously injured. We don't normally go through tissue boxes at our meditations, but at this meeting we did, even though no one attending the meditation personally knew anyone who'd been harmed. Yet far from being depressed by this meditation, we felt better for having done it.

All of us were shaken by the attack. Friends reported on social media that they had been at the finish line where the attack took place. Fortunately for them, they had left before the bombs went off. Others, of course, were not so lucky, and it was the image of one bloodied survivor taken away in a wheelchair that came to me as I brought to mind suffering.

For religious communities, a natural response to a tragedy is to join together in prayer. Having grown up religious, I know from personal experience that prayer can settle one's emotions. But those of us who have left religion — or were never religious to begin with — are not inclined to pray. In such cases, we can turn to meditation to help us deal with suffering. Meditation and the broader practice of mindfulness can shift our feelings from negative to neutral. Mindfulness can be a way of noticing, even amid tragedy, the wonder of being alive.

Before starting the compassion meditation, I didn't know if thinking about suffering would make me less tense or more so. I found, and others did as well, that the practice had a soothing effect. Although thinking about the horror on the in-breath did produce tension, it also produced a sense of connection. Together with the compassion we felt on the out-breath, the overall effect was softening and warm.

People had difficulty cycling between attention to suffering and attention to compassion in sync with the in-breath and out-breath. The images of suffering we'd seen in the media were stark enough that they couldn't be dismissed in a split second. But even if our thoughts were not timed exactly to the in-breath and out-breath, we were able to cycle between awareness of suffering on one hand and feelings of compassion on the other.

Overcoming Compassion Fatigue

The remark "A single death is a tragedy; a million is a statistic" is perhaps misattributed to Josef Stalin.[14] Despite its callousness, this statement captures a quirk of the human mind. The psychologist Paul Slovic has found that the more people we're asked to think about compassionately, the less compassion we feel overall. In fact, Slovic found that compassion fatigue starts to set in as soon as the number of people increases from one to two! That's one reason why charitable appeals often focus on a single "poster child" rather than showering an audience with statistics.

The apparent reason for this phenomenon is that when we relate to people one by one, the brain's emotional circuits are engaged. When more individuals enter the picture, we shift toward a more intellectual, abstract way of thinking.[15] Thus when contemplating a group of people as part of a compassion meditation, it may be best to relate to them one by one rather than all together.

One person spontaneously came up with a mantra, using "broken" on the in-breath and "whole" on the out-breath. I've subsequently found that technique to be useful.

Imagined bodily sensations can be part of this meditation, too. For me, compassion often involves an image of putting an arm around someone to comfort them.

The image of one victim being taken away in a wheelchair made me think about someone close to me who requires a wheelchair. I thought about the struggles she's gone through and whether I've been doing enough to help her and her primary caregiver. Thinking about her made me notice my own slight suffering over this issue and to include myself among those to whom I directed compassion.

Many religious people believe that compassionate thoughts and prayers can affect people at a distance, through supernatural means. As secular meditators, we see meditation as affecting only our own brains and bodies. Meditation changes the world outside our skin only if we follow it up with action. This belief made it all the more meaningful for many of us to donate to fund-raising efforts for victims of the bombing.

It may seem strange to breathe in suffering and breathe out compassion. Wouldn't you want to do it the other way, to breathe in love and get rid of the suffering by breathing it out?

That might seem more logical, but, physiologically, exhalation is more comforting than inhalation. When you breathe in, the muscles of the diaphragm contract, to expand the lungs and draw air in. When you breathe out, the diaphragm relaxes, compressing the lungs and pushing air out. So breathing in actually involves more tension and strain. The physical relief we feel as we breathe out may facilitate feeling warmth and compassion.

You might also wonder whether this is truly a mindfulness practice. Since mindfulness is commonly defined to be a focus on the present moment, the suffering of someone far away might seem to be outside the scope of mindfulness. But a broader definition of mindfulness can include contemplating something that is not in your presence, as long as you are aware of what you're doing. So if you're thinking about the suffering of people whom you've never met and become totally caught up with their suffering to the point that you yourself become traumatized, that might not be mindful. But if you are aware that you are thinking about someone who is not present and also aware of the anger, fear, or other emotional responses that may arise within you, that awareness is mindful.

Laurie's Story

Laurie has been coming to meditations at the Humanist Mindfulness Group for three years. She is a marketing writer and career counselor and also writes fiction. She first attended a Buddhist gathering when she was in high school. "I found the chanting very hypnotic," she recalled. But it was not to her liking overall. "I was a lot more conservative then than I am now, and I just thought it was weird."

In college, Laurie tried transcendental meditation. Instead of helping her feel calm, though, it seemed to bring up emotional issues that made her feel worse. The only instruction she'd received was to repeat a mantra. It didn't help her, so eventually she gave up on it.

Later, she did sound meditation on her own. "I would meditate to music, and I would focus on the music," she said.

She has also done breath meditation, but it doesn't always work for her. "It feels like I'm trying to control my breath too much, and it almost feels like I'm having trouble breathing," she said. "Listening to music or listening to sounds is inherently out of my control. I'm able to let go a little bit more."

Laurie has enjoyed the variety of meditations that we do. One meditation she's found valuable is the *tonglen* meditation, during which one alternatively contemplates suffering and compassion.

"That worked really well for me. The first time we did it was right after the Marathon bombing, so we were all still emotional about that, and that was really helpful," she said. "I got emotional during that meditation, but it was nice to sit there with it and allow that to come out. I did it the following week. It was still a really nice meditation, even though I wasn't quite as emotional that time. I was able to think the words *love* and *compassion* in my head and also feel them."

She has found that it works better in general to be mindful of negative emotions rather than try to repress them. "It's much more helpful to me to allow myself to sit with the anxiety and think about how it feels in my body and allow myself to feel it for a while and accept it. That helps me to let it go. I'm practicing doing more of that in the group."

In this *tonglen* practice, you certainly need mindfulness to be able to shift from thinking about suffering to thinking about compassion. In this practice, you don't get lost in thought but are aware that your thoughts are part of an intentional practice.

Psychologists use the word *metacognition* to refer to thinking about your own thoughts. The Greek prefix *meta-* is distinct from the term *metta* that we use to refer to loving-kindness. Though if you think about your own thoughts with kindness, you could call that *metta* for metacognition!

Questions to Consider

Did you have any difficulty thinking of someone who is suffering?

On balance, did you experience mostly negative or positive feelings during the meditation?

Is there one major cause of suffering in your own life?

Do you experience vicarious trauma through empathy for loved ones who are suffering?

News reports detail the suffering of people all over the world. How do these reports affect you?

Do you feel that sometimes you must distance yourself from suffering in order to protect yourself?

CHAPTER FOUR

Self-Compassion

LOVING YOURSELF might seem narcissistic and conceited. It's certainly easy to poke fun at it. But its opposite, self-abasement, is even less in keeping with humanistic values. The doctrine of original sin, for instance, holds that human beings are wicked by nature and can be redeemed only by believing in supernatural redemption. Humanism arose during the Renaissance with figures such as the Italian poet Petrarch, who asserted that human beings were not completely worthless and could produce valuable secular knowledge.

So it's not self-regard, but *excessive* self-regard that's narcissistic. When a person is successful, we appreciate it if they engage in a little self-deprecating humor. It shows they are keeping things in perspective. So self-love, within reasonable limits, is humanistic. But what's *reasonable?*

In the workshop I took on self-compassion taught by Kristin Neff and Christopher Germer, the first thing that Neff did in her presentation was to distinguish self-compassion from self-esteem. As she defines the terms, self-compassion is a feeling, whereas self-esteem combines positive feelings with an often inflated self-evaluation.

Self-esteem became very trendy a few decades ago, but according to Neff, the results of boosting self-esteem are in, and they're not favorable.[16] The reason it seemed like a good idea was that high self-esteem tended to correlate with success. This connection led people to think that if you could get children to have high self-esteem, they would grow up to be successful.

This view confused cause and effect. Being successful makes you think of yourself highly, with some justification. But thinking of yourself highly, without any regard to your skills and abilities, does not lead to achievement: it may even inhibit it by interfering with the ability to accept constructive criticism that is valuable in learning. Data indicate a rise in narcissism in American society that tracks with rising self-esteem, though the causal relationship is unclear. Contrary to assertions that low self-esteem causes violence, research finds that violence is more common when egotistical people find their inflated sense of self threatened.[17]

In contrast, self-compassion is simply being warm toward yourself. There is no implied comparison with others. As long as you haven't committed a horrible crime, there's nothing wrong with feeling good about yourself. In her book *Self-Compassion*, Neff writes:

> This means that unlike self-esteem, the good feelings of self-compassion do not depend on being special and above average, or on meeting ideal goals. Instead, they come from caring about ourselves — fragile and imperfect yet magnificent as we are. Rather than pitting ourselves against other people in an endless comparison game, we embrace what we share with others and feel more connected and whole in the process. And the good feelings of self-compassion don't go away when we mess up or things go wrong. In fact, self-compassion steps in

precisely where self-esteem lets us down — whenever we fail or feel inadequate.[18]

Comparison and evaluation are zero-sum games. Contrary to what Garrison Keillor says about the children of Lake Wobegon, we can't all be above average. Self-compassion, however, is a positive-sum game. We can love ourselves without taking away from another person's right to be loved.

In the workshop, we were asked to list some of the words we use to criticize ourselves. These could be words like *failure, selfish, stupid*. Then we were asked to imagine a friend saying those same things about us. Would we stay friends with that person?

I agreed that no one in my life would talk to me that way. In fact, when I thought about who would be that harsh, what came to mind was a stand-up comic who picks on people sitting in the front row of a comedy club.

So self-compassion is treating yourself as you would treat a friend. It's not some kind of self-idolatry. It's simply acting toward yourself as you would toward someone who needs kindness.

Self-compassion doesn't mean you can't strive to improve, but it does mean being kind to yourself whether you succeed or not. According to Neff, self-compassion does not undermine people's motivation to succeed. Fear of failure often holds people back from even attempting challenging tasks. An attitude of self-compassion allows people to try things they otherwise wouldn't attempt.

Exercise: Self-Compassion

Compassion meditation can be a formal meditation that one does while seated on a chair or cushion. But you can do it anytime, and you can do it for yourself if you are suffering.

The first step in practicing self-compassion is to notice *when* you are suffering: *when*, not *that*. No doubt you have already noticed *that* you suffer from time to time. This step asks you to be mindful of your emotional state, so that you notice that you are suffering at the time it is happening — in other words, in the moment.

When you catch yourself experiencing a painful thought or feeling, that is the moment when you can practice *tonglen* toward yourself.

Let's say you have a self-loathing thought, perhaps, "I'm a total failure." Rather than get into an argument with yourself about whether the thought is accurate, you can allow yourself to think this thought as you inhale, and feel compassion for yourself as you exhale.

So, in this example, as you breathe in, you'd think:

I feel like a total failure.

As you breathe out, you imagine comforting yourself. This can be done wordlessly. One way to do this is to imagine seeing yourself from the outside as another person would. This other person, seeing you visibly suffering, then puts an arm around you or perhaps holds your hand to comfort you.

Discussion

I think you'll find that this practice of interrupting self-criticism with self-compassion can at least slow down a cycle of ruminations. In moments of self-compassion, you may get enough distance to notice whether your self-criticism contains hyperbole. If you do find that your self-criticism is exaggerated, bring a spirit of self-compassion to that observation, because exaggeration is a habit most of us share.

Self-compassion practice can be fruitfully compared to the techniques of cognitive behavioral therapy (CBT). This is a highly respected form of treatment, with a considerable amount of evidence that it is effective for many individuals. An important aspect of the therapy, as described in the popular book *Feeling Good* by the psychiatrist David Burns, is challenging irrational thoughts. For instance, if you make an overly broad generalization, like "I'm such a loser," you might dispute it by trying to recall situations where you demonstrated poise and accomplishment.[19]

Although CBT has been proved to be valuable, you can't always talk your way out of negative thoughts. For instance, perhaps you really do have a subpar record according to some measure that is important to you. If so, the way to deal with this is not to deny your shortcomings but to insist that, even if you fail more than you succeed, you still deserve warmth, compassion, and love.

In a 2008 paper discussing how cognitive behavioral therapists are incorporating Buddhist techniques, including *tonglen*, into their therapy, Nirbhay Singh and colleagues write, "Some of the newer approaches in CBT, however, are focused less on challenging an individual's irrational or negative thinking and more on changing the individual's relationship to thoughts and feelings through acceptance and mindfulness."[20]

Personally, I find that internal debate over my self-worth sometimes spirals in a negative direction. That is, I lose the debate. And then I might chide myself for that too! Perhaps I'm not applying the technique correctly, but if so, it's hardly foolproof. I find, however, that when I experience a negative thought, if I take a moment to feel compassion for myself, it keeps this cycle of negativity from spiraling out of control.

Self-*tonglen* is not necessarily a panacea. If you really have done something criminal or abusive of another person, then self-recrimination is called for. If it can motivate you to make restitution, so be it. But if you are hurting only yourself, then self-compassion may just be what you need.

Compassion for Anxious Thoughts

I am in general a nervous flyer. I'd tried various mindfulness practices to reduce my anxiety while flying, but they didn't help much. Then, just one week before my wife and I were due to fly to Europe, there was a fatal commercial airplane crash in San Francisco. In the past, that would have started me visualizing my own death in a similar manner. Then I'd feel shame for being fearful, and the negative emotions would just build up in a vicious cycle. This time, I decided to practice *tonglen*, imagining the sickening feelings of being in a crash and then evoking compassion for those who went through the actual experience.

I found that this practice shifted my emotions from a negative state — fear — to a positive state — compassion. Furthermore, it interrupted the vicious cycle of anxiety that would otherwise have built up. I was in a good emotional place for the entire week before my flight. Then, when we did fly to Europe and back, as anxious thoughts arose from time to time, I accepted the slight possibility that the plane I was in might crash. But I shifted my focus from fear to feeling compassion for myself should such an event occur. This short-circuited my normal bouts of anxiety. The flights turned out to be enjoyable and low stress.

Questions to Consider

How warm do you feel toward yourself?

Do you exaggerate your own imperfections?

How socially connected do you feel to others?

Do you feel you are part of a community?

CHAPTER FIVE

Sympathetic Joy

LOVING-KINDNESS IN BUDDHISM is considered to be part of a constellation of four worthy attitudes called the *Brahma viharas*. Besides loving-kindness, the other attitudes are compassion, sympathetic joy, and equanimity.

Sympathetic joy is a curious attitude that is not a distinct concept in American culture. It's the idea that you can derive joy from someone else's joy. Sometimes seeing another person having a good time can make you feel jealous. But if you have a rapport with that person, knowing they are joyful can make you happy.

This experience most commonly occurs within the family. Parents enjoy seeing their kids having fun. And you don't have to have kids to enjoy seeing the smile on a child's face. But when something good happens to one of your peers, envy can kick in. This is especially true if there is any rivalry between you. If your friend gets something that you wish you had, you may have mixed feelings about their success.

Then there's the expression "Misery loves company." When you're down, you feel a little bit better when other people are in the same boat. There's even a term borrowed from German, *Schadenfreude*, that refers to the joy felt on seeing another person suffer.

It's understandable that when you're suffering, you may feel a little bit better knowing you're not alone. But even though it may seem counterintuitive, when you're suffering, if you can focus on another person's joy, you can share it, and that makes you feel better.

Exercise: Sympathetic Joy

Take a walk down a busy street.
Look at people's faces — briefly, without staring.
If you see someone who is smiling, be happy for them.
Notice how it makes you feel about yourself.

Discussion

When I started to do this exercise attentively, I noticed that most people walk with a fairly neutral mask. The people who were really smiling were people talking to other people.

The other people weren't necessarily close friends. Observing people in a business district, it seemed clear to me that the same thing happens with coworkers. Being with other people makes people smile.

This observation reminded me of something that the University of North Carolina psychologist Barbara Fredrickson told me in an interview. "We know from the psychological literature that just interacting with people is by and large pleasant. Even if you are not telling jokes, it's a mood lifter. Interacting boosts mood, more so for some people than others, but pretty much for everybody — unless it's a fight or something."

In fact, when I see someone walking alone with a big smile,

they're almost always wearing ear buds. I presume that listening to music is making them smile.

I hope I'm smiling more as I make these observations.

I think of myself as an introvert. I think meditation appeals to introverts, and most members of the mindfulness group have identified as introverts when asked. Even so, we've found that we enjoy connecting with other people with this similar, introspective orientation.

Most of life is a positive-sum game in which we can all be better off if we play nicely together. Sympathetic joy is a way in which we can share the joys of others and thereby give ourselves a lift.

CHAPTER SIX

Frequently Asked Questions about Compassion Practices

Universal love. Are you serious?

The final step in loving-kindness practice is to expand the circle of *metta* to all beings. This includes all human beings and all animals that are capable of feeling suffering. Cultivating a universal love is a rather ambitious goal.

Wishing well to all beings runs into some logical contradictions. A lion and the gazelle that could be the lion's lunch have a basic conflict of interest: if the gazelle escapes, the lion goes hungry. I presented this conundrum to a couple of Buddhist teachers. Their response was that in thinking of all beings, you're not thinking of individuals, so you don't have to choose between the lion and the gazelle. It's more an abstraction — a feeling of love that you have for everything. It can even extend beyond human beings and animals to plants and inanimate objects. It's just a general, ubiquitous feeling of love.

The intention of universal love — even if it's hard to achieve — is important. Although oxytocin, the brain hormone thought to be responsible for feelings of love and affection, generally encourages prosocial behavior, it can also encourage violence. Specifically, research shows that it promotes defensive aggression, like that of a lioness protecting her cubs. In the human context, oxytocin promotes bias toward one's own group and hostility toward outsiders who threaten the group.[21] It promotes love of "us," which can lead to hatred of "them." The effort to cultivate universal love can expand our concept of "us" to become "everyone" and help overcome hostility among different groups of people.

Restricting love to people of one's own ethnic group, for example, gives rise to bigotry. One recent study has found that in the United States, a lot of discrimination is not due to overt hostility to a different group but favoritism toward people who are like us. People may even think they're not discriminating because they're not motivated by hate but by positive feelings toward people who fit their mold.[22] The problem is that the circle of people they feel positive about is too small.

To be clear, when I say that universal love is possible, I mean that an individual can feel such love toward other beings. I do not anticipate a time when all seven billion–plus human beings feel such love toward each other. Nor do I expect lions to feel love toward gazelles, except in the gastronomical sense.

Surely some people deserve to be hated?

Aspiring to neutralize one's own hostility is reasonable, I think, even with regard to psychopaths and serial killers. Those of us who come from a secular perspective don't believe in metaphysical evil that is the work of a devil. Rather, we consider that some people are damaged human beings who need to be prevented from harming others.

Many people find they can feel compassion for a killer who grew up in underprivileged or abusive circumstances and "never had a chance." Yet even the "overprivileged" who abuse power — you can probably think of political leaders who fit this category — are the products of their genes and their environment.

This thought — that even the worst people are the product of nature and nurture — makes it easier for me to let go of the desire for retribution and look at the situation rationally. Another thought I find helpful is that, if we were created in the image of God, then human beings are a pretty sad lot. However, if we are evolved apes, distant cousins to chimpanzees and orangutans, as seems to be the case, we can feel lucky that things are as good as they are.

Understanding why bad actors do what they do doesn't mean we should let them get away with abuses. It means we should aim to reduce harm without being motivated by hatred, even for oppressors. Wouldn't it be better to focus on love for the oppressor's victims?

Furthermore, it's important to extend our care and concern to people who are unlike us, or even antagonistic toward us. Some of the great crimes that human beings are responsible for have been committed out of love for one's own ethnic or political group. Because people love their own side so much, they want to smash the other side. Being able to see the other side as human and worthy of concern is very important to make sure that we don't become the bad guys, even out of misplaced love.

You don't want me to love mass murderers, do you?

As we cultivate a general feeling of love toward all beings, we need to employ critical thinking to understand how this intention applies in specific situations. I think it's reasonable not to hate mass murderers, but I would draw the line at feeling fondness for them or naively imagining that love will change their hearts.

Feeling love toward dangerous individuals may, in fact, be dangerous. Scientists find that feelings of love dampen activity in brain areas that make negative judgments about other people. Researchers in Belgium found that subjects who were given oxytocin in a nasal spray took fewer pains to secure a questionnaire containing confidential information about their sex lives compared to subjects who were given a nasal spray with no active ingredient. This was measured by having the subjects submit the questionnaire for computerized scanning either in a sealed or unsealed envelope. Leaving the envelope unsealed was interpreted as a measure of the subjects' trust in the researchers' promise not to peek at the information.[23]

In other words, love counteracts fear and builds trust. This may be good in many situations. But the fight-or-flight response evolved for a reason. If someone is trying to kill you, getting the hell away from them is a proven survival strategy. Trying to get through to them emotionally is not a surefire approach.

As a rule of thumb, when people are verbally abusive, it is appropriate to practice *metta* toward them. After all, if you are skilled at practicing *metta*, which includes generating warm feelings toward *yourself*, those warm feelings can counteract and protect you from hostile words thrown at you. But they won't protect you from a punch or a bullet, so practicing *metta* toward someone who is threatening you with violence may not be a good idea.

Aren't you just talking about forgiveness?

That depends on how you define forgiveness. Often, when you forgive someone, the slate is wiped clean. The shift to emotional neutrality I'm suggesting is perhaps closer to "Forgive, but don't forget." This approach is particularly appropriate when the offender continues to do harm. By forgiving, you let go of negative emotions that eat at you. But if you forget, you may leave yourself vulnerable to repeated injury.

I'm suggesting that we distinguish between emotional and cognitive elements in our reactions to events. We can let go of emotional judgments and the desire for retribution while holding on to hard-earned wisdom that can help us prevent future suffering (including our own).

An Unlikely Case

In her 2005 book *Unlikely Angel,* Ashley Smith relates how empathy for a murderer may have saved her life. Smith was taken hostage by Brian Nichols, the now-convicted "Atlanta Courthouse Killer," who was on the run after shooting a judge, a deputy, and a court reporter. He told his hostage that he'd been in court to be tried for rape, a charge he indignantly denied. Smith listened to him and allowed herself to empathize with his sense of having been wronged. She also shared with him her own history of brushes with the law and her struggle with drugs. Eventually, he let her go and surrendered.[24]

Empathy is no foolproof elixir. It's best not to approach a dangerous individual unless you're trained in such matters. Of course, once a killer or other harmful person has been incarcerated, compassion indicates that we should see that their confinement is humane and as conducive to rehabilitation as possible.

Won't unbounded loving-kindness make me an easy mark?

One outcome of *metta* meditation appears to be increased trust. I've been in correspondence with the authors of an as-yet-unpublished study in which students were randomly assigned to groups that were taught either *metta* meditation or mindfulness-of-breath meditation. Before and after the four-week meditation courses, participants played something called the trust game. In this game, participants are given real money they can keep. If they entrust a partner with some money, and that partner proves trustworthy, both can gain additional money. But if the partner exploits their trust, they can lose money. Researchers found that among students who had to move first in the game, those who had learned *metta* meditation shared 40 percent more money, indicating a higher level of trust. Students learning mindfulness of breathing, in contrast, grew no more trusting over the four-week period.[25]

It would be good to have a practice that can make us more

loving and trusting. This raises the question, though, of when it's wise to use this practice. After all, not everyone is trustworthy.

The neuroscientist Paul Zak of Claremont Graduate University has also used the trust game to study students, in this case nonmeditators. Zak found that as many as 5 percent of the participants siphoned off all the money their partners entrusted them with. Anyone who trusted these people was making a mistake. From testing participants' blood samples, Zak found that those who took advantage of their partners were more likely to show signs of abnormality in the way they process oxytocin, one of the hormones associated with feelings of empathy. Zak does have a pungent term for these nonreciprocators: "bastards."[26]

Ideally, we would like to be able to trust people without falling prey to scam artists. If *metta* works by stimulating oxytocin release, one relevant finding is that oxytocin improves "mind reading." That is, people given oxytocin, compared to those given a placebo, are better able to gauge the moods of others from their facial expressions.[27] Thus, if you can better empathize with people, you may be more aware of when a person is hostile.

Another study that employed the trust game found that oxytocin makes people more trusting except when there are cues that the other person might not be trustworthy; among the cues that made people wary was that the other person was in the marketing field.[28] It seems that *metta* inclines us to give the benefit of the doubt to people we judge as neutral. But as long as we stay mindful, we can pick up on signs that such a person might actually be untrustworthy.

Done properly, *metta* practice can neutralize ill will toward difficult people while keeping us mindful of the potential harm they might do. However, achieving this balance can be tricky for beginners. "When people start doing loving-kindness, they sometimes say, 'I love anybody, I don't lock my doors anymore. I don't lock my car. Everybody is invited to my house.' This is stupid, right?" the Buddhist teacher Christiane Wolf said. "You have to use common sense."

Thus, it's up to you to decide whether you wish to act kindly toward a stranger. If you choose kindness, don't assume that it will be reciprocated. But even if it isn't, you may find that being kind provides its own reward in the form of the feelings that it inspires within your own brain.

Psychopaths and Empathy

Not everyone has a normal experience of empathy. In his book *The Science of Evil*, the scientist Simon Baron-Cohen (cousin of the comedian Sacha Baron Cohen) writes about some of these people. Some are harmless. People with autism spectrum disorder have difficulty processing emotions. However, in general, they don't harbor ill will toward others and aren't deliberately harmful. There is another class of individuals who have difficulty feeling empathy but apparently enjoy feelings of power and domination over others. They are called psychopaths.

The psychologist Robert Hare developed a psychopathy checklist to identify people in this category. As he wrote in his 1993 book *Without Conscience*, it's characteristic of psychopaths that although they lack empathy for others, many of their other emotional faculties are intact, and in fact they can be very flattering and charming.

Hare roughly estimates the number of psychopaths in North America at two to three million, or slightly less than 1 percent of the population. Despite the terms *psychopath* and *serial killer* being almost synonymous in popular culture, most psychopaths are not violent. Although psychopaths do make up about 20 percent of the prison population, Hare's best guess is that no more than 1 in 20,000 psychopaths are serial killers.[29]

Hare mentions the case of Jack Abbott, a prison inmate with literary ability who came to the attention of the writer Norman Mailer. Mailer helped Abbott with the publication of a book, and Abbott was paroled from prison. Shortly after his release, Abbott got into an argument with a waiter at a New York restaurant and stabbed the waiter to death. He was returned to prison, and in subsequent interviews made clear that he thought the waiter's death was no loss to the world.[30] His lack of remorse suggests an inability to empathize with his victim or the victim's loved ones, even after sufficient time had passed to allow Abbott to reflect on his actions.

Recently, the UC Irvine neuroscientist James Fallon has written that his own brain shows strong signs of psychopathy. He admits to being an "asshole" but says he's not a violent person. He argues that it takes both a predisposition to psychopathy, which he has, and a harsh or abusive environment, which he did not experience, to create a harmful individual.[31]

There is someone who has hurt me so much that I don't think I can think about them with loving-kindness. What do you suggest?

The idea in *metta* practice is to generate *positive emotional momentum* by first thinking about people you care for and then redirecting those feelings toward people you don't care for. By definition, the neutral person is someone who doesn't inspire strong feelings. So thinking about the neutral person shouldn't lessen this momentum. But thinking about a "difficult" person may generate negative feelings strong enough to overwhelm your feelings of *metta*.

That is why it's best to start with a slightly difficult person — say an irritating coworker — rather than the most difficult person in your life.

The goal here is to shift your feelings toward this person so that you neutralize your ill will. It's not necessary or even advisable to try to shift your feelings so that you cherish them or even want to be in the same room with them. By neutralizing hostility, you can think about this difficult person without your emotions clouding your judgment.

Why should I love someone who doesn't love me back?

Even among people of goodwill, one cannot be certain that kindness will be reciprocated. People are busy and stressed. One solution is not to crave reciprocation. Unrequited love, whether romantic or platonic, can be a source of suffering. But loving-kindness, extended unconditionally, can be its own reward.

One thing you'll realize from the experience is that *love comes from within.* That may sound like a cliché, but it's absolutely true. The brain is what generates feelings of love, and you can learn to generate those feelings.

We tend to think that someone has to love us before we can feel love. But in fact we can feel love toward others whether or not it's reciprocated, and we can feel love toward ourselves. And it feels good.

People can be confused about this idea, because when you love someone and they don't love you back, it can hurt. The cause of the suffering here, though, is not feeling love toward this person but clinging to the desire that they love you back. If you love the Eiffel Tower, do you feel upset that it doesn't reciprocate your love? Of course not. If you can love a person without requiring that love to be reciprocated, you can avoid the pain of unrequited love.

Isn't this love stuff just for privileged people who don't have any problems?

Quite the opposite. These insights, derived from Buddhism, originated as a way of dealing with suffering 2,500 years ago, when people were far more exposed to scourges such as famine and disease. So they are indeed meant for people with problems.

The one caveat is that learning to shift one's feelings, while ultimately refreshing and energizing, can be demanding at first. Mental exercises are like physical exercise in that you may have to invest some effort before you see benefits. In fact, mental exercises actually are subtly physical, because the source of our thoughts and feelings is a bodily organ, the brain. It's estimated that the brain burns 20 percent of the energy used by the body.[32] This energy is provided by glucose or blood sugar. So these practices will be more challenging if you have not eaten or slept well.

What scientific evidence is there that metta practice works?

The psychologist Barbara Fredrickson did a study of *metta* meditation and then a fifteen-month follow-up on those who learned the meditation to see if it stuck.[33] She told me: "Loving-kindness meditation does shift people's daily experiences of emotion in a significant way, and it doesn't just affect their feelings of love and closeness, or trust or compassion. We found that across ten different positive emotions, people showed an upward shift in their feelings of pride, in their feelings of interest and curiosity, in their feelings of amusement." Its effects are not limited to the period of formal practice. "It's not just what people are feeling while they're meditating. It's what they're feeling the rest of the day," she said.

Fredrickson's emphasis on positive emotions is somewhat different from the views of Buddhist teachers I interviewed. Narayan Helen Liebenson of the Cambridge Insight Meditation Center emphasized that the *intention* toward loving-kindness was important, whether or not it translates into feelings. "That loving feeling might accompany the intention. If that happens, wonderful. You really want to be in the body when you're doing *metta*," she said. "You want to let the intention affect your body, let the intention infuse your body."

Fredrickson puts more emphasis on feelings. "Our data so far suggests that positive emotions are a really important mediator. And yet the real psychological action of *metta* meditation doesn't come while you're meditating. It comes while you're interacting with the world. Working on that intention then changes what people's motives are when they see people and interact with them in their daily life. They approach it with more warmth and good-will and care and concern."

Fredrickson's original study of *metta* meditation found bene-fits among participants taking a seven-week meditation class. In her follow-up study of participants, Fredrickson found that one-third maintained a regular meditation practice of some sort. "The peo-ple who were still practicing were doing better than all the others, and they weren't doing better beforehand. That was the real key. It wasn't like they were the 'happy people' for whom loving-kindness came easily." She said her results indicate that *metta* meditation does not simply produce a change in a person's short-term mental state; it also develops durable aspects of personality that some psycholo-gists refer to as "traits" but that she prefers to call "resources" be-cause they can accrue or wither over time. Such long-term changes suggest the brain may be rewiring itself in some way, as generally occurs when a person learns a new skill.

Interestingly, Fredrickson told me she first became interested in *metta* not because she was particularly interested in Buddhism but because she was looking for a tool that would help her study positive emotions in general. "We actually had done some inter-vention studies prior to working with loving-kindness meditation that were all just colossal failures," she said, so she was excited to find that *metta* produces long-lasting benefits.

"People got better and better at it with practice, which speaks a lot about the prospects of mind training. It is a skill that people are getting and developing," she said. "So many other interventions in positive psychology wear out — go south — after a little bit."

How does metta *work in terms of brain chemistry and neuroscience?*

Love for one's children makes sense in evolutionary terms, but it's a bit surprising that we can extend love more universally. It turns

out that the mammalian social-bonding system works in a suffi-
ciently general manner to allow broad application. The actions of
the hormones oxytocin and vasopressin are key in social bonding,
as demonstrated by the work of the biologist Sue Carter.[34]

Studying different species of vole, a mouse-like mammal,
Carter observed that the male prairie vole mates for life with his
female partner and helps care for the offspring. In contrast, the
male of a related species, the meadow vole, abandons his mate and
progeny. An important difference between the two species is in
the number of oxytocin and vasopressin receptors in their reward
system — a key part of the brain that helps motivate animals (including us). When a male prairie vole interacts with his mate and
offspring, the flow of oxytocin and especially vasopressin in his
brain spurs activity in the reward system, which means he likes it
and wants to do more of it. With fewer receptors for these hormones in the reward system, the male meadow vole finds parental
activity to be of little interest.

Additional evidence for the role of oxytocin and vasopressin
comes from studies involving genetic engineering. The neuroscientist Larry Young and colleagues succeeded in getting nonmonog-
amous meadow vole males to become monogamous by injecting
them with vasopressin receptor genes from monogamous prairie
voles. Mice that were genetically engineered to lack a functioning
oxytocin system, by contrast, have a sort of amnesia for social
relationships. Unlike regular mice, they treat mice they've met
before like strangers.[35] However, oxytocin and vasopressin have
other biological roles in mammals in addition to social bonding,
and other avenues that promote social bonding may exist that do
not involve these hormones.

The neuroscientist Paul Zak has extended the study of oxytocin in social bonding to our own species. "What we've shown
is that oxytocin release is stimulated by acts of kindness or trust
by complete strangers," Zak told me in an interview. "The feeling

people get when their brains release oxytocin is one of empathy or emotional connection."

In his 2012 book, *The Moral Molecule*, Zak writes that the action of the oxytocin system underlies "the Buddhist concepts of metta (loving-kindness) and karuna (compassion)."[36] I asked Zak if oxytocin release would occur when you engaged with a person in your imagination, as happens in *metta* meditation. Although he had not studied that question specifically, he noted that one of his most effective methods of eliciting oxytocin release is to show subjects a video about a child who was dying from cancer. So oxytocin can be released when one has an imagined experience of emotional connection: it seems likely that this would occur in positive situations as well as tragedies.

A considerable amount of research shows that imagining doing something activates many of the same brain circuits as actually doing it, though with less intensity. Brain scans have shown, for instance, that the brain activity of people imagining playing the piano is similar to that of people actually playing it. The primatologist Frans de Waal and the neuroscientist Stephanie Preston argue that this is a general feature of the brain that is true not just of overt actions such as playing the piano but also of emotional acts like empathy.[37] If they are correct, then imagining an emotional connection with another person should activate the same brain systems as when the other person is physically present.

Barbara Fredrickson is studying the specific question of whether oxytocin is released when people practice *metta* meditation. Her understanding of the mechanisms of social connection makes her think it is. "Based on the animal literature, based on the limited human literature, there is every reason to believe that's likely to be the case, which is why we're going after it," Fredrickson said.

By definition, people feel positively toward benefactors. But when we contemplate the neutral person in *metta* practice, why don't our feelings quickly snap back to neutral? What accounts for the carryover or emotional momentum that makes us feel kindly toward a neutral person? It may be due to the persistence of oxytocin and vasopressin. A team of European researchers led by the neuroscientist Kjell Fuxe notes that these hormones — like other small-molecule peptide neurochemicals — are released in quantity from cells to diffuse relatively slowly throughout the brain, unlike chemical neurotransmitters at synapses, which are transferred in a fraction of a second.[38]

"There is roughly a twenty-minute window in which, once your brain has released oxytocin, we've shown in experiments that people are basically much nicer to each other, give much more to charity. They behave in ways that are very prosocial even with strangers," Paul Zak told me.

Thus, it is plausible that the warmth and benevolence produced in *metta* meditation promote the release of oxytocin and vasopressin in the brain. These neurochemicals might continue to circulate for several minutes afterward. If you shift your thoughts toward a neutral person during this period, you may find, to your surprise, that you *like* this person. When you then shift your thoughts toward a difficult person, the neuropsychological momentum of oxytocin, and related thoughts and feelings, may continue — unless your aversion to this person is so strong that it triggers the release of neurochemicals that counteract oxytocin.

The brain chemicals released when we contemplate a benefactor, then, seem to have a spillover effect that makes us feel more kindly toward everyone — for a matter of minutes. But if *metta* meditation made us loving only during the formal practice itself, and we snapped back into unkind habits immediately thereafter, it wouldn't be all that valuable. Oxytocin has a long-term impact on our nervous system, according to Zak. "We are laying down memory tracks using oxytocin on who is safe, trustworthy, and kind. These memories are being rehearsed each time we have a positive interaction, and so it can lead to us being kinder to more people more of the time. Practice is the key to activate this effect," Zak said.

PART TWO

Finding
Inner Peace

CHAPTER SEVEN

Mindfulness of Breath Meditation

THE FIRST PART OF THIS BOOK focuses on *metta* — cultivating an attitude of kindness toward loved ones, neutral people, and even difficult people. In mindfulness, we cultivate an attitude of kindness not just toward people but toward *anything* that's happening right now. Mindfulness is often defined as nonjudgmental attention to the present moment. But according to the Buddhist teachers I've spoken to, nonjudgmental doesn't mean apathetic. Rather, it's an attitude of indiscriminate kindness or *loving* attention.

"*Metta* is one of the qualities or aspects of mindfulness," Narayan Helen Liebenson told me. "When you look at an experience, it's warm, it's nonjudgmental." Nonjudgmental should not be confused with neutrality, however. "We want to see everything with eyes of loving-kindness," Narayan said.

Metta practice is one aspect of mindfulness. The other is *attention to the present.* That means focusing on what is going on right now, not only in your surroundings but also inside your body, including your brain. And you try to notice it with kindness.

If you're worried about something that might occur tomorrow, or ruminating about something that happened to you five years ago, you're not focused on the present moment. However

— and this is a subtlety — if you step back and notice that you're thinking about next Friday, that noticing *is* mindful, because you're noticing a thought occurring in the present moment. But having raised this subtlety, I'm now going to drop it until much later in this book, because it's a little too meta (with one *t*), too self-referential, like a hall of mirrors. If you're just beginning the practice of mindfulness, trying to be mindful of thoughts about the future is not the place to start.

Mindfulness is a good skill to have. You don't have to be present at all times: this is not a commandment. But it is a practice that is widely useful. We all have experience in being distracted; it's good to know how to focus.

For this meditation, we're going to be mindful of our breath. That means paying attention to the breath with a kindly attitude. This is a narrow, or concentrated, form of mindfulness, in that we're focusing on one particular object — our breath.

There are other things going on right now that we could notice if we wanted to, but we're not going to be mindful of them. Mindfulness is about the present moment, but the focus can shift from a wide angle of noticing all sensations to a narrow focus such as concentrating on our breathing.

For most people, breathing has a neutral feel to it, neither positive nor negative. But when concentrating on the breath, negative thoughts may arise about how you're breathing, so an attitude of kindness comes in handy.

If you find being mindful of the breath is difficult, you're in good company. Actually, I find it difficult. I don't connect all that well to the tactile or kinesthetic feeling of my body as I breathe. If anything, I become more engaged with the sound of my breathing. For many people, however, paying attention to the breath works really well, so it's a good place to start.

One problem people have with this meditation is that they try to control their breathing. Breathing is one of the few functions of the body that can be done either automatically or voluntarily. When you fall asleep, you still breathe, even though you're unconscious. When you're awake, you can choose when to breathe in, when to hold your breath, and when to breathe out. For one or two breaths, that's fine. But when people try to control their breath for an extended period, they sometimes feel anxiety. This is because most of us don't have conscious knowledge of how to regulate our intake of oxygen and release of carbon dioxide. Excessively rapid or deep breathing can even lead to hyperventilation and a panicky feeling.

For the meditation, it's best to let the body do the breathing by itself. Just notice passively what your body is doing as it breathes in and out.

Exercise: Mindfulness of Breath Meditation

Allow 20–40 minutes for this exercise. If you are meditating on your own, you may wish to use a timer so that you don't have to check to see how much time has passed, which can disrupt your concentration. If you are a beginner, twenty minutes is a good time to set aside. If you've been meditating for a while, you can set aside a longer time to meditate.

Find a cushion or a chair that allows you to sit up fairly straight. Make yourself comfortable. Take off your shoes if you wish. Loosen any tight clothing.

You may wish to place your hands in your lap or on your thighs.

Close your eyes, or if you prefer, keep them open but lower your eyelids and soften your gaze. Even if your eyelids are closed, you can reduce tension by softening the eye muscles.

If you find yourself falling asleep during the meditation, it can help to open your eyes.

Although you don't want to control your breathing during the meditation, you can start off by taking a deep breath or two.

When paying attention to the breath, people often find it useful to narrow their focus on one aspect of the breathing cycle. You might focus on how your belly rises and falls, or you might notice the breath passing in and out of the nostrils.

A good way to start is by silently counting your breaths. You can count each inhalation and exhalation up to five and then start over.

Let's do that:

(breathing in) One. (breathing out) One.
(breathing in) Two. (breathing out) Two.
(breathing in) Three. (breathing out) Three.
(breathing in) Four. (breathing out) Four.
(breathing in) Five. (breathing out) Five.
(breathing in) One. (breathing out) One.
And so on.

You don't need to keep counting your breaths throughout the entire meditation, but it can be a good way to start.

You may prefer to focus solely on the exhalations. Once you're comfortable with that, you can focus on the inhalations too. Once you're comfortable paying attention to both the exhalations and inhalations, try paying attention to the stage in between when your lungs are temporarily at rest.

If you can focus entirely on your breathing for five breaths, that's quite an achievement.

You don't need to breathe in any special way, though as you

meditate, your breathing will likely become deeper and more regular.

If you notice your mind wandering, don't try to suppress those thoughts. Instead, treat them kindly, like the difficult person in the *metta* practice. Then return to the breath.

When the allotted time is up, open your eyes. Notice the sights and sounds around you. Has your perception of sights or sounds changed in any way?

Discussion

One of the benefits of breath meditation is that it quiets the mind. When I first heard the expression *quiet the mind*, I didn't know what it meant. How could your mind be quiet? I'd never experienced such a thing.

But as I meditate, I do find that my inner voice becomes quieter — more like a whisper — and can be entirely silent for ten or twenty seconds at a time. This is longer than you might think, and it's very peaceful. I'll discuss later on how this happens, but for now the important thing to remember is that you don't have to push your thoughts away. Just by meditating, they are quieted naturally. Of course, sometimes a person just can't settle down, and the thoughts don't cease. But if you've changed your attitude toward these thoughts, and can look on them with kindness, you're making progress. With practice, the inner chatter is likely to become less insistent.

When your mind does quiet, words are not within easy reach. Without language, it's hard to think about the past or the future. You are anchored in the present moment. And if you can't think about the future, it's hard to worry about the future.

Sometimes mental images pop up that take you out of the

present moment. But if your inner voice is quiet, you're less inclined to apply judgments to them. They arise and disappear, but they don't stimulate a further train of thought.

People often report a heightened awareness of sights and sounds when they emerge from meditation — I do. It probably won't happen the first time you meditate but may well occur if you meditate once a week for twenty minutes over, say, four weeks.

Tom Clark is the director of the Center for Naturalism, which promotes a science-based worldview. He described his own experience with meditation to me:

> I find there is a heightening of sensory awareness, certainly. Things do become more vivid and clear.... You are in a heightened state of receptivity, of sensitivity to what's going on in your surroundings because you're not focused on your thoughts so much.... When you get up after meditating, you're still somewhat in this mindset. With the thoughts slowed down and awareness heightened, you are more sensitive to just about anything that comes your way. That will last for a while — minutes to a half hour, an hour longer after meditating.

For several years, I've presented meditation videos online at a site called *Seeing the Roses*. The inspiration for that name came when a friend of my wife's asked me to show her how to meditate. I led her in a twenty-minute breath meditation. It happened to be Valentine's Day. When she opened her eyes after the meditation, her glance fell on a vase full of red roses her husband had given her. She told me that she saw them differently on coming out of the meditation. They were more striking, more beautiful than before.

My Story

Back in the 1980s, when I first encountered meditation, I was quite scornful. Having moved to California from the East Coast after graduate school, I was looking for a house to share. I checked out one in Berkeley, where I was told that one of my prospective housemates was in the backyard meditating. I thought this was typically Californian. I never imagined I'd be doing it myself.

I didn't move into that house, but I did have an experience in the Bay Area that changed my life. Over a period of eight years, increasingly intense eyestrain had been making it difficult for me to work. It got to the point where I applied to be certified as visually handicapped. I saw eye doctors — including one who suggested my vision problem was psychosomatic, a diagnosis I rejected indignantly.

Finally, I was referred to an ophthalmology specialist at the University of California San Francisco Medical School. He told me that my eyes were fine but that I'd become hypersensitive to minor eye sensations. A thought struck me. My overprotective mother had frequently warned me about reading too much, even shouting, "Stop reading! You'll be blind by the time you're thirty." Nearing thirty, I believed I was going blind. It was a self-fulfilling prophecy.

I decided then to accept the eye sensations I experienced as nonthreatening. Within forty-eight hours, my eye pain faded, and I was able to function normally again. It felt like a miracle — like being born again — and if it had happened at Lourdes rather than at UCSF, I might be Roman Catholic today. My healing occurred at the medical campus where the neuroscientist Howard Fields and colleagues demonstrated how the placebo effect works: the body generates its own pain-relieving opioids when tricked into expecting pain relief from a placebo. I suspect that the physicians there were well informed about the effect of mental attitude on pain. Although I had not heard of the concept of mindfulness at that point, my recovery is quite consistent with the idea that the way we respond to an experience, rather than the experience itself, is what produces joy or suffering. Many years later, I interviewed neuroscientists and physicians for magazine articles on how mental attitudes affect feelings of pain and suffering.[39]

This experience shook me and opened my mind. The Y in San Francisco where I went swimming offered a class in meditation. Even though the eye condition had been resolved, I realized that my neurotic and stressed nature might cause difficulties again, and it would be good to learn to relax.

The meditation class at the Y was entirely secular — just like another exercise class. The instructor showed us how to breathe diaphragmatically, so that the belly expands, rather than breathing shallowly into the chest. She also taught us to count as we breathed in and out. That was pretty much all we learned, but it was a good start.

After the class was over, I thought I'd like to keep up a meditation practice. So I checked out a local Zen center, but the bowing and chanting had a religious feel to it that I found off-putting. I didn't go back. After moving back to the East Coast, I meditated less and less, in part because I didn't know anyone else who did it. Eventually, thinking that I needed to connect with other people who meditated, I signed up for a class at another Zen center, but that didn't really take either.

In 2006, a passenger sitting near me on a plane turned out to be a teacher at Naropa University, a Buddhist-affiliated university in Boulder. He and I talked for the rest of the flight. He recommended the Cambridge Insight Meditation Center, which he said had more of a secular feel.

I went to the center and liked it. I learned many things there that I'm sharing here. Insight meditation is a Westernization of the Theravada tradition, which is the main form of Buddhism in parts of Southeast Asia, including Thailand, Burma, and Sri Lanka.

A little later I got involved with the humanist community. I attended a conference at Harvard in 2007 called "The New Humanism," featuring speakers such as the novelist Salman Rushdie. After the conference, I got to know the leader of the Humanist Community at Harvard, Greg Epstein, and became part of a humanist discussion group.

Greg, who had studied Buddhism in Taiwan, encouraged members of the community to form what we now call the Humanist Mindfulness Group. Eventually this group merged with a similar group that called itself "secular Buddhist." Although I was not the founder of either group, I have been the main organizer of the combined group for the last few years.

It used to be that scientifically oriented people (like me) rolled their eyes when they heard about meditation. Now there's enough published research that many nonreligious people accept that meditation has value and can be done in a secular manner.

When we started our group, we focused mostly on breath meditation. In trying to bring contemplative practices to a secular audience, however, I've come to view *metta* as an easier entry point. When I talk about love and friendliness, people know what I mean. Furthermore, humanism defines itself as having a social mission — to be of service to other human beings. A practice that cultivates loving-kindness clearly connects to that goal.

Questions to Consider

Conditions such as hay fever or asthma can create anxiety as you attempt to follow the breath. Do you have any physical conditions that interfere with easy breathing? If so, another type of meditation, such as ambient sound, may be a better fit for you.

When you are not meditating, do you normally breathe shallowly into the chest, or do you breathe deeply, into the abdomen?

Do you often find that thoughts fill your head and are difficult to turn off?

Did you notice changes in your body during the meditation?

Did you notice changes in your thoughts or the frequency of them during the meditation?

Did you feel relaxed or restless as you came to the end of the meditation?

CHAPTER EIGHT

Ambient Sound Meditation

WHEN WE LEARN TO MEDITATE, we generally begin in a quiet environment. But we can meditate even in a noisy environment. Our group meets in Harvard Square, which is often noisy, with loud, heavy traffic and sometimes even a marching band passing right outside.

Mindfulness is paying attention with a sense of kindness and without judgment. Calling something *noise* already implies a judgment. When I interviewed Reya Stevens, who leads classes on Buddhist approaches to illness, she made this point. "Is it noise or is it sound?" she asked me. "Inherent in the word *noise* is your aversion to it. You're labeling it as unpleasant."

With the sounds we think of as noise, it's *how* you pay attention that's important. Mindfulness is awareness with an open, accepting, friendly, or even loving attitude. If you hear the rumble of a truck, don't think, "Ugh! A truck." Don't even think, "Truck." Notice the hiss, the rumble, the whine, the screech, and the whoosh. Notice whether the sounds are high or low in pitch, whether they are short and sharp or drawn out. Notice as the sounds rise in volume and as they fade out. When you do this, what was irritating becomes energizing.

You can treat a noise like the difficult person in loving-kindness practice. Just as you shift your perception of a difficult person, you can shift your perception of a difficult sound.

If there's one spot that is almost proverbially loud, it's a subway train. Yet in his book *Breath by Breath*, the insight meditation teacher Larry Rosenberg describes mindfulness in that environment: "In my life around Cambridge and Boston, I frequently ride the subway. People carry on about how wearing such encounters with mass transit are and how depressing. But I often ride long distances and use the trips as occasions to meditate: no special clothes, no cushion, no bells or incense, just a guy sitting on the subway. I bring attention to the present experience and live those moments. It isn't depressing at all."[40]

I sometimes meditate on the subway. The roar of the train and the screeching of the brakes are just sounds — more things to pay attention to. Sure, I sometimes listen to music on an iPod. But it's good to not be dependent on electronic devices. You really can enjoy the present moment in almost any situation you find yourself in.

Mindfulness of Sirens

Mindfulness can help you take pleasure in just about any sound — even those you may consider to be noise. This was quite a revelation to me when I attended a workshop a few years ago led by the Buddhist teacher Jack Kornfield.

He told a story about someone who lived near a fire station. When meditating, this fellow would focus on his breath. Every time a siren went off, however, it would interrupt his meditation. It was quite a struggle. Then he learned that although it is common to focus on the breath during meditation, there are many other objects one can focus on. If a siren demands your attention, you can focus on that. Eventually, this guy became so good at meditating on sirens that he missed them when things got quiet.[41]

Exercise: Sound Meditation

Allow 20 minutes for this exercise. Get into a comfortable sitting position, just as you would do for a *metta* or mindfulness of breath meditation.

Take a deep breath or two to relax. After that, there's no need to follow your breath.

Now, start paying attention to sounds. If indoors, you may hear creaks, rustling, and sounds from electrical appliances. Listen for sounds drifting in from outside. In this exercise, there are no bad sounds.

If meditating outside, you'll probably hear a cornucopia of sounds — wind, birds, traffic.

When you hear a sound, don't merely note it and shift your attention away. Try to listen to the sound for its entire duration. Notice how it rises and falls.

In a lull during which there are no sounds, you can shift your attention to your breath — perhaps to the sound of your breathing. But if other sounds do arise, turn your attention back to them.

Discussion

Building on the theme of loving-kindness, you can think of noise as that "difficult person." By cultivating kindness as a general practice, when noise does occur, you can turn to it with affection or even gratitude. It doesn't have to break your meditation.

I can now meditate to traffic sounds with ease. The sound I find most intrusive is the human voice. It's not a question of whether the voice is pleasant or unpleasant. Rather, it's that if the words I've overheard are intelligible, they can set me off on a train of thinking.

Even there, however, I'm making progress. Some time ago, my wife didn't realize I was meditating and turned on a Red Sox game. At first I was irritated by the sound and thought of getting up from my chair to shut the door. Instead, I tried listening to the announcer, to the tone of his voice, and to the words, but without processing them — letting them go in one ear and out the other, with just a slight pause to notice them. It worked. I found that much of the time I was able to listen without reacting, though mention of one player, Dustin Pedroia, started me wondering how he was progressing in his recovery from an injury and when he would return to the lineup. After I caught myself being distracted, I was able to shift back to what the announcer was saying in the present moment. I found I could meditate in the presence of language without getting hooked by the language.

Pat's Story

Pat teaches at a local university and has been coming to the Tuesday night meditations regularly for the last year. She found out about the group on Meetup.com, where we are listed as the Cambridge Secular Buddhists. Pat was interested in Buddhism but somewhat wary.

"Putting the adjective *secular* in front of it reassured me," she told me. "Buddhism is a religion. There is a lot to like about it. It's not the religion I grew up with. I grew up Roman Catholic. Buddhism was refreshing because it wasn't Roman Catholicism. But anything too supernatural or dogmatic makes me a little uncomfortable."

Pat adds that she doesn't consider Buddhism to be all that dogmatic, but it does have certain beliefs that are not necessarily supported by solid evidence. To be among people with a thoroughly secular outlook has raised her comfort level with these practices. "This was a need that I didn't realize I had until it was met," she said.

Mindfulness practice helps her cultivate both attention and self-compassion. "With sound and breath meditation, there is this idea that when you're listening to ambient sound or your breath and you get distracted, instead of letting that distraction take over and warring with the distraction and saying to yourself, 'Oh, I'm being distracted, I shouldn't be distracted. Bad, bad, bad meditator!' you just set it aside and gently bring it back to the traffic noise or the breath."

She likes that we start with a silent meditation, but also that afterward, people discuss how their meditation went. "It's nice to know what the range of possibilities is, and we do it in a very non-judgmental way," Pat said. "It's an icebreaker in a way, even if you don't have much to say. It's just a way of getting people talking."

After that, we open the conversation up to "joys and concerns" and encourage people to talk about whatever important is going on in their lives. This is different from the sort of conversations that occur in many other humanist venues, which are often focused on a political or philosophical issue.

"I'm not interested in a purely academic conversation, and you know me, I am an academic," Pat said. "There is a lot of inner work — psychological, emotional, and relationship work — that comes up in our conversation.

"What's really important to me is that it's conversation with heart," she said, citing personal issues that come up, like people's sometimes conflicted relationships with their parents.

"For me it's really about the people," she said. "Sharing vulnerabilities leads to connection."

Even though mindfulness practice is about being compassionate and accepting, Pat said that it has had a surprising benefit. "This sort of practice is helping me be more assertive, because I'm getting more *skillful* at being assertive. I can assert myself without it being this big fraught deal." While she doesn't seek conflict, she can deal with it now. "I'm not shaken by it as much as I used to be."

Pat finds the mindfulness practice she is developing to be especially helpful in her dealings with students in her freshman writing seminars. "Basically, I'm nurturing the next generation. That's my orientation," she said. "There is an emotional side to writing. You're vulnerable." It can hurt to hear that your writing is no good, Pat said, which is why she tries to be compassionate when giving feedback.

"I have to be very mindful and present," she said. That's especially so during one-on-one writing conferences she has with students.

"Sometimes, frankly, a student comes in and I get annoyed or bored. The annoyance or boredom — I have to set it aside," she said. "The breath meditation and the sound meditation, and doing *metta* at home or on Tuesday nights, raises my baseline of tolerance, compassion, and the ability to orient myself toward the other person rather than coming in with a prejudice that they're annoying or boring.

"I'm getting more skillful at identifying the precursor of annoyance, and stepping outside of it and being present for the real conversation," she said. "In general, my students and I have a good rapport, and that's why it's so important to me not to let the inevitable moments of annoyance get out of hand."

Pat said she appreciates that our group tries to encourage a collegial atmosphere — kind of like a seminar — rather than a hierarchical teacher-student relationship. She has even begun to lead some meditations, especially one that has become her favorite — mindfulness of sound.

Questions to Consider

Did the meditation go as you expected, or were there things that surprised you?

What sounds did you find surprisingly tolerable or even enjoyable?

Were there any sounds that you couldn't easily tolerate?

How did you deal with the silences?

Did you incorporate elements of other meditations, such as loving-kindness or breath meditation?

CHAPTER NINE

Mindfulness of the Body Meditation

THIS CHAPTER INTRODUCES a guided meditation called the body scan. This is a form of mindfulness in which we use a specific technique to pay attention to the various parts of the body. It is a key element of the Mindfulness-Based Stress Reduction (MBSR) program created at the University of Massachusetts Medical School by Jon Kabat-Zinn. The MBSR program is a secular mindfulness program that borrows from Buddhist practice; the body scan was adapted from a Burmese Buddhist practice.[42]

In this meditation, you slowly pass your attention over the body, from bottom to top. When I say slowly, I mean really slowly. You'll be amazed how long we spend on the foot.

If there's a part of your body that's in pain, you may be concerned that paying attention to it will make it worse. Paying attention to a painful body part in a nonmindful way, with a sense of aversion, thinking "Make it go away," can indeed make it feel worse. But if you pay attention to a troublesome region with an attitude of kindness, you may find that the meditation takes the edge off the pain a bit. Just as you can have *metta* toward a difficult person, you can have *metta* toward a body part that's acting up. The physical sensation may still be the same, but because your emotional reaction to it is different, it's not as disturbing.

Even though this is a very physical meditation, sometimes emotional issues come up. The Brown University neuroscientist Catherine Kerr has studied meditators who practice the body scan. She told me, "Many people who were in the study found the body scan challenging, and they also found it had very strong, unexpected emotional effects." That's because our emotions are based not solely in the mind but also in the body. Although this is most evident in our facial expressions, where our muscles often show our emotions, we also display emotion through our posture. You can tell when someone is standing proudly or slumping over in sadness. When we feel things in our gut, we have a tightening in the stomach and intestines. Then there's the "sinking feeling" we have when we receive bad news. When people feel fear, their bodies tremble. When they are nervous, they experience tensing and agitation of the muscles.

Most people find the body scan meditation to be very relaxing. But if disturbing emotions arise as you're contemplating a particular part of the body, it may be best to skip quickly to the next part.

Let's give it a try.

Exercise: Body Scan

Allow 20 minutes to one hour for this exercise. This is a guided meditation. Because the instructions are long, if you are meditating on your own, you may want to record the exercise below and play it back as you meditate. It doesn't make exciting reading, but if you listen to and follow the instructions, it can be very rewarding. Take at least twenty minutes to move your attention through the body, but go even more slowly if time permits. Take at least two full breath cycles for each body part.

If you do this without a voice to guide you, it's good to use your own inner voice to name each body part, mentally labeling it as you rest your attention on it.

Make yourself comfortable. Take off your shoes. You may want to loosen your belt. You can do this meditation in a chair, but you may want to do it lying down, perhaps on a carpet. It's probably best that you close your eyes.

Start off by taking a couple of deep breaths. Just relax.

Now focus your attention on the little toe of your left foot. If you've never done this before, you may have difficulty feeling the little toe. If so, try to wiggle it to see if you can gain awareness of that area.

Just put your attention into that little toe.

Take a couple of breaths.

We're going to bring that same level of loving attention to each body part, all the way up to the crown of the head. It is not necessary to consciously relax a body part; simply paying attention to it will often accomplish this.

So from the little toe, now shift your attention to the adjacent toe of the left foot.

Take a couple of breaths.

Now, if you can feel them, try the third and second toes. Personally, I can't feel these toes as distinct entities, but I can feel the two of them together.

Now, shift to the big toe.

Remember to take a couple of breaths each time you shift attention from one body part to another.

Sweep your attention back and forth over the five toes you've passed through.

Now, on to the ball of the foot.

To the arch of the foot.

Now the heel.

Now sweep your attention across the entire sole of the left foot. The sole should be nice and relaxed.

Let your attention slide up to the instep.

To the ankle.

When you're ready, shift your attention to the lower left leg. Let's start with the shin.

Sweep your attention round to the calf muscle. Let your attention flow all the way up the calf.

Now, let your attention flow up to the inside of the knee.

Around to the kneecap.

Now up to the quadriceps — the front part of the thigh.

And around to the rear, muscular part of the thigh.

Let the attention flow up to your butt. (When referring to private regions of the body, use any name that makes you feel comfortable.)

Now, we'll shift over to the right side of the body. Take a nice breath and shift your attention to the right side of your butt.

Now sweep it around to the front, to your pelvic region.

Now, let's do the right leg, starting at the thigh and working down. Give it just as much time as you gave the left leg.

Shift your attention to the right thigh, starting with the top of the thigh.

Now down to the bottom, muscular part of the thigh.

To the inside of the knee.

To the outside of the knee.

To the shin.

To the calf.

Down to the ankle.

Instep.

Forward to the big toe.

Successively to the other toes. All the way to the little toe.

Back to the ball of the right foot.

The arch.

The heel.

Now sweep your attention all along the right sole until it is nice and relaxed.

When you're done, sweep your attention back up your leg and all the way to your belly. As you breathe in and out, does your belly move up and down?

Now, sweep your attention up to the breastbone.

To the center of the upper chest.

To the area of the left breast.

Over to the area of the right breast.

Up to the collarbone of the right shoulder.

Now over the right shoulder, resting your attention on the shoulder blade.

Down the right arm to the biceps muscle.

Underneath to the armpit.

Down the triceps muscle on the outside of the arm to the elbow.

To the inside of the elbow.

The inside of the forearm.

The outside of the forearm.

Down to the wrist.

The back of the hand.

The palm of the hand.

Out the thumb all the way to the tip.

Out the index finger all the way to the tip.

Out the middle finger.

The ring finger.

The pinky.

Now sweep your attention back up the arm again to the shoulder blade.

Now, to the upper part of the back, just below the neck.

Down the back to the mid-back.

To the lower back.

If you're finding an area that's painful — and sometimes the lower back can be tight or sore — don't dwell on it. Keep shifting your attention after taking a couple of breaths.

Sweep up the back to the left shoulder blade.

Down the left arm to the biceps.

Down to the armpit.

Down the triceps to the outside of the elbow.

The inside of the elbow.

The inside part of the forearm.

The outside of the forearm.

The wrist.

Back of the hand.

Palm.

The right thumb all the way to the tip.

The index finger all the way to the tip.

Middle finger.

Ring finger.

Pinky.

Now sweep back up the arm to the shoulder and to the lower part of the neck.

Remember to breathe mindfully.

Up to the nape of the neck.

The back of the head.

The left ear.

The left cheek.

Down to the jaw. Let the jaw drop, keeping your lips together.

Shift your attention down to the throat.

Now up through the jaw to the tongue. Pay mindful attention to the tongue — especially the base of the tongue toward the back of the throat.

Now move your attention to the right cheek.

To the right eye. Soften the eye.

Now to the nose.

To the left eye.

Up to the forehead.

Across the hairline to the crown of the head.

Now, sweep your attention from head to your toe to see if any part of the body has become tense again. Just give it a little more attention, take a breath or two, and let it go.

Discussion

After this meditation, your body should be pretty relaxed. It may be surprising that simply paying attention to your muscles can relax them.

I find the body scan to be very effective when I devote enough time to it. Sometimes I rush through it quickly to relieve the muscular tension that I feel. That can help, but to get the full benefit, you have to spend time on it. Twenty minutes is about the minimum to get a good effect. Longer is better.

The Body Scan and Chronic Pain

The neuroscientist Catherine Kerr suggests that the body scan may affect the "body map" in the brain, sometimes called the *homunculus* and humorously depicted as a little man inside the head. The brain's body map is actually a distorted version of the body's surface. Some areas, like the chest, are relatively insensitive to touch and disproportionately small in the body map. Others, like the lips, are very sensitive and disproportionately large. The homunculus, when depicted artistically, has the lips of Angelina Jolie, the chin of Jay Leno, the hands of Arnold Schwarzenegger, and the chest of a ninety-eight-pound weakling.

Kerr cites evidence that when we pay more attention to a body part, the corresponding region in the homunculus swells. For instance, people who read Braille have more sensory territory devoted to the index finger.[43] Similarly, people who experience chronic back pain may have more neurons monitoring the back. Picture a distorted map in which a state's size is based on the electoral votes it possesses, so that New Jersey looks bigger than Alaska. The distorted sensory map of a person in chronic pain similarly enlarges the body parts in pain. Paying equal attention to all areas of the body using the body scan meditation may reduce this distortion. "Our theory is that meditation actually fine-tunes that ability to maintain sensory equanimity," Kerr told me.

Questions to Consider

In one of his short stories in *Dubliners*, James Joyce describes a character who "lived at a little distance from his body."[44] How close do you live to your body?

Are there any parts of your body you are uncomfortable with?

Is it possible that you could consider them old friends?

In the meditation, were there parts of the body that you had difficulty accessing?

Doug's Story

Doug is a scientist and meditator whose work includes scientific research on meditation. Doug told me that he first became interested in meditation as a way of dealing with insomnia.

"I was having problems falling asleep. I was actually up in the middle of the night one night, not falling asleep, and remembered that Human Resources had sent out a blurb talking about stress reduction. They were advertising the very next day that Herb Benson was giving a little lunchtime workshop," Doug said, referring to the author of *The Relaxation Response*.

Doug discussed the workshop with a colleague, who invited him to participate in her brain-imaging study of the effects of meditation. The study involved participating in an eight-week mindfulness-based stress reduction class. "I saw immediate progress in terms of my sleeping," Doug said, "and it seemed to help out with a lot of other things as well."

Doug said he found it really helpful to listen to a guided body scan meditation on a recording before going to sleep. "You start at your toes. You work from your toes all the way up to your head, just being aware of bodily sensations. The first time that I tried that, I got up to about my waist, and then I fell asleep."

He laughed. "I thought, 'This is just a gimmick.' But the next night, the same thing happened. It doesn't happen that way every night. I certainly still have problems falling asleep, but they are dramatically better."

After the eight-week class, Doug started going to meditations at the local Insight Meditation Center and has even gone on some long retreats. Regarding the first retreat, he said, "The first couple days, I was freaking out. I was going, 'What am I doing here?'" Doug said, "Then I really settled into it....I got to places where the actual sitting meditation was very, very deep."

Doug tries to apply his mindfulness practice outside the meditation hall as well. "Sitting practice is only part of the practice. I don't see the sitting practice as the end goal of anything. It's like going to the gym and working out. What I practice for is so the rest of my waking moments, I can be happier, more mindful, a more present person and live my life in a way that's consistent with my values."

CHAPTER TEN

Face Meditation

I'D LIKE TO INTRODUCE YOU to a practice that I personally find to be the best way to quiet the inner voice. When your inner voice is quiet, when words are not at the tip of your tongue, it's difficult to think about the past or future. You are anchored in the present moment. The practice turns down the volume of self-condemning thoughts.

The practice is to relax — deeply relax — the muscles you use while speaking. Surprising as it may seem, your inner dialogue involves the muscles of speech. Inner speech is not contained entirely within the brain. It leaks out into the peripheral nervous system and causes the muscles of the tongue, lips, and voice box to tense slightly.

Edmund Jacobson, a twentieth-century American physician and researcher, was the first to discover the connection between the inner voice and the muscles of speech. Jacobson worked with engineers from Bell Laboratories to invent some of the earliest devices to measure electric charges in human muscles.[45] These devices enabled Jacobson to make objective measurements of muscular tension. Using his inventions, he was able to correlate subjects' reports of inner speech with heightened electrical activity and muscular tension in the muscles used in speech. He also found that when you relax the muscles used for speech, including muscles controlling the tongue, your inner speech becomes quieter.

I'd known about Jacobson's work for some time, but I didn't connect it to meditation until I read a book by the meditation teacher Anna Wise. Although Wise's 2002 book, *Awakening the Mind*, is in many ways too New Age for my tastes, one of its insights has been extremely valuable to me. She writes:

> When people think, they have a tendency to talk to themselves. Even if you're not aware of the subvocalization, your tongue will feel tense — ready — when you are thinking. You may experience this as a gentle pulling on the back of the tongue, or you may not feel at all. If you relax your tongue *completely*, you cannot talk to yourself. Therefore, it is more difficult to think....*If you take nothing else away from reading this book, you will have gained enormously from this one practice.*[46]

Paul Lehrer, a professor of psychiatry at Robert Wood Johnson Medical School in New Jersey, was a student of Edmund Jacobson. "He was a real down-to-earth engineering type. He didn't like anything that sounded mystical," Lehrer told me. Jacobson himself was a student of Walter B. Cannon, the Harvard Medical School physiologist who first identified the fight-or-flight response.

In 1978, in the fifth edition of his book *You Must Relax*, the long-lived Jacobson wrote of his test subjects: "When requested to imagine counting to ten or to recall the words of a poem or something they had recently said, most of them stated that they had sensations in their tongue and lips and throat as if they were actually speaking aloud, except they were much fainter and briefer. Upon relaxing the tongue, lips and throat muscles completely, most of them stated that imagining or recalling the numbers or words was discontinued."[47]

When I asked him, Lehrer agreed that a meditative technique that relaxed the muscles of speech would quiet inner speech. "Thinking takes place with the whole body. It doesn't just take place in the brain," Lehrer told me. "Almost any kind of thought involves muscle tension. The primary spots for thought-related muscle tension would be, as you mentioned, the muscles of the mouth and the vocal cords but also the muscles of the eyes."[48]

The speech muscles tense in a way that is specific to the sound being subvocalized. For instance, thinking the consonant p results in tension in the lips, whereas thinking of a t tenses the tongue. Because of this specificity, engineers at NASA's Ames Research Center have developed inner-speech recognition sensors that can be placed under the chin and voice box. A commercial prototype was one of the winners of *Popular Science* magazine's Invention Awards for 2009.[49]

Perhaps you buy the idea that the vocal cords are somewhat involved with thought. But what about the eyes? Although, in general, we think in words, it's possible to think in pictures too. Jacobson found that when people construct images in the mind's eye, they tense their eye muscles. To test this finding, with your eyes closed, try to recall the living room of the house you grew up in. Look around it in your mind's eye. As you scan the room, do you notice your eyes moving under your eyelids? Mine do.

Jacobson found that relaxing or softening the eye muscles quiets the visual imagination. According to a 2007 paper by Lehrer:

Verbal components of undesired thoughts, such as those of phobias and worries, can be eliminated by relaxing the speech muscles (tongue, lips, jaws, throat, and cheeks).

The eye muscles are the focus for eliminating the visual imagery of thoughts. When the eye muscles are totally relaxed, one does not visually perceive anything; the eyeballs must move in order for visual perception or visual imagery to occur. Thoroughly relaxing all of the muscles of the body can bring all undesired mental processes to zero.[50]

When the facial muscles are relaxed to this degree, in fact, one tends to fall asleep. Jacobson even wrote a book based on these findings called *You Can Sleep Well*. If you are trying to meditate, of course, you don't want to relax quite that much. However, if you are troubled by negative visual imagery during a meditation, try softening the muscles of your eyes to inhibit visual thinking. To be clear, this refers to images that pass across your mind's eye while you are awake — for instance, images of paperwork on your desk at work. If you doze off during a meditation, you may see random, dreamlike images. If you find yourself falling asleep while meditating, it can help to open your eyes slightly.

Now, let's give this a try.

Exercise: Face Meditation

Allow 30 minutes for this exercise. Before we can learn to relax the muscles of speech, we have to familiarize ourselves with these muscles. So let's start with some speech exercises to become more mindful of how we produce speech.

If you are doing this exercise as part of a group, it's okay to laugh. If you are doing it on your own, you'll probably want to do it in private so people don't laugh at you.

1. Notice how your tongue contributes to speech. Say out loud, "Nick Norris nibbled nachos." Now, think the same words. Do you notice tension in the back of your tongue?

2. Notice how the throat contributes to speech. Place the fingers of one of your hands gently on your throat, in the area of the Adam's apple. Say out loud the vowels: A, E, I, O, U. Notice the tension in your throat as you say the vowels. Now, lower your hand. Try this again by only thinking the vowels. Do you notice any tension in the throat?

3. Let your jaw drop. Notice how your tongue and lips relax too.

4. Scan through your face, relaxing any remaining tension in the speech muscles. Relax the throat by paying gentle, friendly attention to the area of the Adam's apple, which covers the voice box or larynx.

5. Once your muscles are relaxed, try to speak out loud without tightening your muscles. Your speech should sound garbled. If it is articulate, the muscles are still tense.

6. If your outer speech is garbled, check your inner speech. It should be fairly inarticulate as well. Try thinking the words of a famous poem or speech, for instance Hamlet's "To be or not to be." If your inner voice sounds incoherent, you're doing it *right*.

7. So that you can do this practice in public without embarrassment, bring your lips gently together. If you keep your upper and lower sets of teeth apart, that should prevent clenching and will keep the tongue relaxed.

8. You may find your tongue wavering or floating inside
    your mouth. If you find this distracting, try resting
    the tip of the tongue gently on the roof of the mouth.
    You can place it on the palate, just behind the teeth or
    a little further back.

9. If you wish, notice how eye muscle tension contrib-
    utes to visual imagery. With your eyes closed, visual-
    ize a scene with some movement — a baseball player
    hitting a pop fly that sails upward, or a kid bouncing
    up and down on a trampoline. Do you notice any
    movement of your eyes under the lids? Now, relax
    the cheeks and the muscles around the eyes. Feel
    them soften. Can you still visualize the pop fly sailing
    upward? Doesn't the image slip away as you soften
    the eye muscles?

10. Let's get into a meditation. If noticing tension in your
    face is proving to be a challenge, let that be the focus of
    your meditation. Treat it like a body scan meditation
    from the neck up, paying friendly attention to all the
    muscle groups of the face or neck. If you find it easy
    to relax the face, then do any meditation you prefer. If
    you notice mental chatter, switch from your standard
    object of meditation (e.g., breath or sound), and do a
    quick scan of the muscles of your face. Let them go
    limp. Then return to your regular meditation.

Discussion

When we did this as a group, about half the people reported that
their inner voice quieted more quickly than in other meditations.
One attendee mentioned that he'd come up with a practice of
changing his inner voice by making it sound like a high-pitched
cartoon character. Doing that certainly makes you take it less

seriously. You can also try making your inner voice speak in a deep baritone. When I do this, I notice that I have to tense the muscles in my throat to lower the pitch. This is a dramatic reminder of how the inner voice depends on the muscles of speech.

Another way I've found to quiet the inner voice is to rest the tip of my tongue on the roof of my mouth. In the *Vitakkasanthana Sutta*, an ancient text of the Pali canon, the Buddha recommends this practice as a last resort in order to stop unwanted thoughts. I've found little scientific research on it, but my guess is that any tongue position that interferes with out-loud speech also interferes with inner speech.[51] Try singing "Yankee Doodle" with your tongue pressing against the roof of your mouth and you'll see what I mean.

We know that movement of our facial muscles feeds back to affect our feelings and possibly our thoughts. One study found that saying the *e* sound in *cheese*, which forces the facial muscles into the position of a smile, is experienced by people as pleasant, while the German *ü* sound, as in *München*, is a downer, even for Germans. Researchers have also found an unexpected side effect of Botox injections, which are used to reduce facial wrinkles by paralyzing facial muscles. Injections that paralyze the muscles used in frowning not only make it harder to express sadness; they also make it harder to feel sad.[52]

Facial feedback seems to be a specific, well-studied example of a general phenomenon. Tensing or relaxing muscles anywhere in the body can have an effect on emotions. Charles Darwin noted the connection as far back as 1872 in one of his lesser-known books, *The Expression of the Emotions in Man and Animals*. He wrote: "Most of our emotions are so closely connected with their expression, that they hardly exist if the body remains passive." He also observed, "The free expression by outward signs of an emotion intensifies it. On the other hand, the repression, as far as this is possible, of all outward signs softens our emotions."[53] The only dispute I have with Darwin's statement is in the use of the word *repression*. Actively trying to repress an emotion can create tension. To relax facial and other muscles, what's called for is gentle, loving attention.

To get technical for a moment, the signals from the brain to the muscles run in a loop. The brain sends nerve signals down to the muscles to tell them how to move. However, the muscles also send signals back up to the brain, telling them what they did, in a process called *proprioception*. There is good evidence that this feedback loop runs in a continuous cycle at a frequency of ten times a second or more.[54]

It appears that when the muscles become less active, activity is inhibited in the brain areas that the muscles are connected to. In an experiment where people watching emotional videos were told to keep their faces motionless so as not to interfere with dummy electronic sensors, they reported feeling less emotion than when they were free to move their faces.[55]

Facial feedback may thus explain why relaxing the muscles of outward speech quiets inner speech. Self-talk is accompanied by low-level activation of the muscles of speech. Relaxing those muscles inhibits inner speech.[56]

Questions to Consider

Were you able to bring conscious awareness to the muscles that produce speech, including those around the voice box?

Were you able to relax them?

Did they revert to a tense state?

Is your face normally tense or relaxed?

Is your jaw usually set or loose?

Do you have a characteristic expression that inhabits your face?

Do you think it's hokey to "put a smile on your face"?

CHAPTER ELEVEN

Mantra Meditation

WE'RE GOING TO DO SOMETHING slightly different now — a mantra meditation derived from Hindu rather than Buddhist practice. As humanists, we're not particularly tied to Buddhism. We're interested in any practice that works. We're willing to try practices derived from Hinduism or any other religious traditions if they are useful and can be secularized. In fact, even though the state of the art in secular meditation has moved in a more Buddhist-influenced direction, the first popular secular meditation was derived from Hindu practice.

The scientific study of meditation started with Herbert Benson, a cardiologist at Harvard Medical School and the author of the 1975 book *The Relaxation Response*. Benson was concerned about the effects of stress on heart disease. The fight-or-flight stress response clearly has evolutionary value as a way of allowing us to escape predators and other dangers. But when frequently activated, it can overtax the body and lead to heart attack and stroke.

The stress response and what Benson calls the relaxation response are opposing actions of a part of the nervous system that affects our inner tissues, or viscera. In a talk in 2010, Benson recounted, "We found early in our work that meditation led to a response that looked exactly *opposite* to the fight-or-flight response, and it was done in the very room at Harvard Medical School in which the fight-or-flight response was discovered by Walter B. Cannon sixty years before."[57]

The form of meditation that Benson presents in *The Relaxation Response* is a secular form of transcendental meditation. The original transcendental meditation (TM) was a somewhat secularized version of traditional Hindu religious practice, but it was not entirely free of what most skeptics would think of as supernatural belief. For instance, the TM movement sponsored large group meditations in the belief that they would lower crime rates in surrounding communities through psychic effects alone.[58]

Transcendental meditation first gained popularity in the 1960s as a result of interest among the Beatles and other pop figures. As Benson tells it, some practitioners of TM approached Harvard Medical School, hoping to be studied. Benson figured there was nothing to lose by checking it out.

Benson made various physiological measurements of transcendental meditators and found promising results, particularly with regard to lowering high blood pressure. Meditation was not, as some argued, a form of sleep. Benson identified the elements of TM that he thought were critical to producing beneficial effects:

1. A quiet place to meditate
2. Something to focus on — a word or phrase to repeat or an object to gaze on
3. A passive or accepting attitude
4. A comfortable posture

TM makes use of a mantra — a word or phrase repeated over and over again. Some mantras used in TM are said to have religious significance, but in Benson's secularized version, any word or phrase can serve. He suggested using the word *one*.

Meditators would repeat the word *one* over and over again silently and in conjunction with breathing — for instance, saying "one" with each exhalation. Using this technique, people would reach a state of meditative calm in ten to twenty minutes.

Benson was a pioneer in creating a secular meditation program in a medical context. In recent years, his mantra-based program has been surpassed in popularity — at least among academic researchers — by MBSR. However, recently Benson has collaborated with geneticists who have shown that mantra meditation activates genes that regulate and maintain the mitochondria, the powerhouses where cells produce their energy.[59]

The simplest mantra is a single word of your choice, like *one*, that you repeat over and over again. Personally, I find using a single word boring. I prefer to use two words — one for the in-breath and one for the out-breath.

In our group, we've started blending Benson's approach with a technique suggested by James Austin, a neurologist and Zen meditator who has written a number of books on the neuroscience of meditation. In perhaps his most accessible book, *Meditating Selflessly*, Austin recommends a technique of counting breaths that transitions into a kind of mantra.[60] So our mantra meditation is a kind of hybrid of mantra and breath meditation.

Exercise: Mantra Meditation

Allow 20 minutes for this exercise. Before you start, pick two words or short phrases to use, one for the in-breath and one for the out-breath. They can be meaningless, or they can be words that remind you to be mindful. For instance, the words *just* and *this* can remind you to pay attention just to the present moment. *Just* and *love* can keep loving-kindness present in your mind. Using *I* on the in-breath and *we* on the out-breath can help you expand your circle of concern from yourself to others.

In the guidance for the mindfulness of breath meditation, I suggested you start by counting your breaths. We'll start this meditation doing something similar.

So, get comfortable, relax, and take a few deep breaths.

Now, start by using the word *just*, and a number. Match these to the breath. Say the words silently to yourself. Extend the length of the word to match the duration of an inhalation or exhalation. For instance, "just" would actually be "juuuuust."

Just... (inhale)
One... (exhale)
Just... (inhale)
Two... (exhale)
Just... (inhale)
Three... (exhale)

When you're comfortable with this, you can transition to using your mantra, for instance:

Just... (inhale)
This... (exhale)
Just... (inhale)
This... (exhale)
I like the mantra *one love*.
One... (inhale)
Love... (exhale)

Whatever mantra you choose, this technique is a nice way to combine mindfulness of breath with a mantra. If you're having trouble coordinating the mantra and the breath, let go of the breath and just focus on the mantra.

Discussion

The first time I used *one love* as a mantra, I had an excellent experience. I repeated *one* on the in-breath and *love* on the out-breath. Then — and I'm pretty sure this was subconscious priming — it occurred to me to change *love* to *heart*. At first I resisted, because in the traditional meditation, the mantra is not supposed to change. But I went ahead and changed it.

I then recognized that I was picking up on dimly remembered song lyrics. I synced my breaths to the refrain, so that four inhalations and four exhalations matched the opening line of the song. And since those were the only words from the song that I knew, I kept cycling through them. Later on, I looked up the lyrics and realized they were from the song "One Love/People Get Ready" by the reggae star Bob Marley. The song is actually a religious hymn, but the refrain is fine for humanists.

Repeating this mantra put me in mind of universal love. As I kept doing it, I felt tingly all through my body — except my neck, which can be stubborn that way. Everything was so relaxed. I felt the way I do when I'm with someone and feel a real sense of communion.

Later, as we went around the room to discuss how the meditation had gone, I got choked up. Embarrassed, I tried to disguise my feelings as laughter. But it was partly laughter and partly something more emotional.

Questions to Consider

Were you able to draw out the mantra so that it covered
    most of the breathing cycle?
Did the mantra's meaning generate any thoughts or emotions?

Did you let go of the mantra after a while and just follow the breath?

Do you have any personal mottos?

Are there any lyrics, poems, or quotations that could serve as mantras for you, either in whole or in part?

CHAPTER TWELVE

Frequently Asked Questions about Mindfulness

What does being nonjudgmental really mean in the context of mindfulness?

Mindfulness is often defined as nonjudgmental attention to the present moment. But the word *nonjudgmental* can mislead, because it may seem to indicate neutrality or apathy. In fact, in the Buddhist tradition at least, it's meant to be warmer than that. There's equanimity to it, because you're taking everything in without clinging to the things that are consistent with your goals or pushing away the experiences that conflict with your goals. But you can have a generally warm attitude of *metta* toward everything.

The Buddhist teacher Christiane Wolf told me that this quality of *metta* is sometimes being forgotten as mindfulness becomes more secularized. "There are more and more people teaching mindfulness who don't understand and who don't live the compassion and loving-kindness part of mindfulness. Especially with this whole movement in the psychotherapy world, a lot of people are teaching mindfulness more like an attention skill. If you do that, compassion can easily fall under the table."

Even though our project here is to secularize Buddhist practices, I don't see a need to strip *metta* out of mindfulness. Compassion is also an aspect of humanist philosophy. Attention training by itself can be used for good or ill.

The word *nonjudgmental* can mislead in another way too, because it doesn't mean you shouldn't make rational decisions. It's really about not making *emotional* judgments. A few years ago, I interviewed Shinzen Young, a mindfulness teacher who is noted for his work with people in chronic pain. Young says that while mindfulness is often defined as "nonjudgmental awareness," more precisely it's a question of equanimity.

"Nonjudgmentalness can be a factor of equanimity, but equanimity is a broader concept," he told me. Equanimity does not mean passivity. When you have a physical injury, or even the kind of pain that might indicate a heart attack, instead of panicking, you can mindfully apply good judgment and do what needs to be done. "You can have equanimity with the physical sensations, the thoughts, and the feelings," Young said, "while you take objective action."

It helps to distinguish between judging as thought and judging as feeling. Judgment in the sense of using reason and logic is not a problem. The kind of judgment we're trying to get away from in mindfulness is the feeling of aversion, the feeling that you're trying to push something away. Trying to reject negative feelings compounds the negativity. Paradoxically, when you accept negative feelings, they tend to go away on their own.

What do you mean by "inner chatter"?

Inner chatter is one of the major distractions that interferes with mindfulness. We can divide the inner speech that goes on inside our heads into two types. The first is inner speech that is directed toward a goal. For instance, as I write these words, I am forming the words and phrases inside my head moments before I type them into a laptop. This type of inner speech is pretty useful, and I can't imagine how I could write a book without it. Would my fingers, unguided by thoughts, produce anything but gibberish? Arguably, I'm being mindful as I write these sentences, because I'm aware of my thoughts and finger movements.

The other type of inner speech is the stream of chatter that seems to go on without purpose — what is often referred to as the "stream of consciousness." Scientists find that inner speech is produced spontaneously — without reference to any previous event — by the brain's default mode network.[61] It is referred to as *default mode* because this is what the brain does when it's not doing anything purposeful — when it's not paying attention to anything. When your mind wanders, it flits from thought to thought until you catch yourself and perhaps wonder, "How did I get to thinking about that?"

When your mind wanders, inner speech arises spontaneously. Scientists aren't sure why this occurs, but it does allow you to think about new problems and perhaps come up with solutions. Daydreaming by itself is not necessarily a bad thing. But if you are chewing over scenarios that cause you to worry, it's useful to know how to quiet those thoughts.

One way to quiet the inner chatter of a wandering mind is to pay attention to something. Attention to anything — the breath, ambient sound, a flower — shifts the brain out of this default mode. As long as you are paying attention, this network is deactivated and does not produce spontaneous inner chatter. That is one way that meditation quiets the mind. This could be called a top-down approach because the executive areas of the brain, which are activated when we pay attention, inhibit the chatty default mode network.

Another way that meditation may quiet the mind could be called a bottom-up approach. Relaxing the muscles of the tongue, lips, jaw, and throat quiets inner speech. That's because of a feed-back loop between the areas of the brain that produce speech and the muscles that articulate speech. When these muscles are deac-tivated, it appears that the areas in the central nervous system that respond to their feedback also become less active.

This could account for the persistence of inner quiet after the conclusion of a meditation, when a person is no longer focusing attention on an object of meditation, like the breath. The quieting of inner speech during a meditation causes the muscles of speech to deactivate. At the conclusion of a meditation, these muscles may remain in a relaxed state for some time, inhibiting the resur-gence of inner chatter.[62]

Simply put, how does mindfulness relieve stress?

Think about it this way. What do you worry about? Most likely, it's something that could occur in the future, not something that is happening in the present moment. If something horrible were hap-pening right now, you wouldn't be reading a book, would you?

In addition to worrying about the future, we tend to ruminate about the past. We have a whole lifetime full of past moments, and some of them were negative. We can chew over them, and experience the pain all over again, even though we can't change the past. Although in certain circumstances it's a good idea to consider past mistakes to make constructive changes for the fu-ture, research indicates that rumination often is not fruitful and can lead to depression.[63]

Most of the time, the present moment is okay. And if you focus on the present moment, which is what we do in mindfulness, then you are focusing on something that is okay, so you won't be stressed about it.

But what if something bad *is* happening right now? There is an old story of a Buddhist monk walking through a forest who encounters a ravenous tiger. The monk runs, but as he nears the edge of a cliff, he stumbles. Over the cliff he goes. Before he tumbles too far, he manages to latch on to a vine. Whew! He looks up. The tiger is peering down at him. He looks down. The ground is a dizzying drop below. He looks in front of him and sees the vine tearing away from its roots. Then he notices a wild strawberry plant growing out from a crevice in the cliff. With his spare hand, he reaches out and eats the fruit. Wonderful![64]

I thought of this story when my wife and I were canoeing in Quebec and got into a bit of trouble. Paddling along the steep-walled Malbaie River gorge was spectacular — until we tried to turn around. Our first attempt to turn the canoe around failed. I was confused. Trying again, I realized we had been canoeing with the prevailing wind and were now struggling against it. At some risk of capsizing, we managed to turn the canoe around and head back. But with a sinking feeling, I realized we were making no progress. The wind seemed to be holding us in place as we paddled, or even pushing us backward.

Eventually, we started to make slow progress. Still, I was concerned we might capsize, and even if we made it, we wouldn't return to the boat rental area until after it had closed. Yet even as we grappled with an unpleasant situation, I thought it would be a shame not to enjoy the spectacular scenery. The story of the monk and the strawberry came to my mind. I was determined to notice and enjoy the canyon walls even as my tired arms struggled to paddle. We eventually arrived back safely before closing time.

Even when the present is difficult, it may be possible to find moments of pleasure and serenity amid the chaos.

Do mantras work differently from other forms of meditation?

Mantra meditation may have its own unique way of silencing inner speech, which has to do with the way working memory operates.

Working memory is a special type of short-term memory in the brain: it's the memory we use to deal with the present moment.

If a man introduces himself to you at a cocktail party and then two seconds later you don't remember his name, it's because this piece of information was never transferred from working memory into longer-term memory. When you want to remember someone's name you might repeat it a few times: "Mike, Mike, Mike, Mike." This repetition keeps it in working memory long enough for it to be transferred to other types of memory.

A well-regarded model of working memory was put forward by the British psychologist Alan Baddeley. It includes an element called the articulatory loop, which contains a very short-term memory for sounds that can be reinforced by silent rehearsal — by saying the same thing over and over again in your inner self-talk.[65]

One piece of evidence for this model is that some individuals with a certain form of amnesia can keep thoughts in this very short-term memory and keep repeating them for a substantial period. But if they get distracted, those thoughts are gone, and they never get into the individuals' long-term memory.[66]

It appears that we have only one audio channel in working memory. As a result, hearing other sounds can interfere with our inner speech. This is illustrated in an episode of *The Simpsons* in which a character is playing loud music. Homer Simpson comes in and complains it's so loud that he can't hear himself think. Just when you're wondering what idea Homer could possibly have, Homer thinks to himself: "I want some peanuts."[67]

This interference doesn't have to come from outside. Psychologists have found that if subjects repeat an irrelevant syllable while memorizing verbal information, it interferes with understanding of the information. Similarly, one recommended technique for treating insomnia is for the aspiring sleeper to silently repeat the word *the* every three seconds. It's hard to keep up a train of thought when your working memory is clogged by an irrelevant word. The authors who recommend this technique note that it works best in blocking internal chatter that has little emotional weight.[68]

Essentially, this technique is the same as repeating a mantra. The verbal repetition makes it hard to have coherent verbal thoughts about something else. To the extent that you can prolong your mantra to match the entire length of an in-breath and the entire length of an out-breath, then stray verbal thoughts can sneak in only during the pauses in between. You could say that a mantra jams the verbal part of working memory.

I asked Paul Lehrer about how mantra meditation works. "It does block the ability to think other thoughts. You can't think a mantra and worry at the same time. You're using the same brain pathways," Lehrer said.[69]

Isn't paying attention boring?

Actually, paying attention is fun. This may be counterintuitive, because it probably evokes a memory of a teacher shouting, "Pay attention!" and your not wanting to. The problem with school is that kids are often there against their will. But if you see a child absorbed with watching a crawling ant or a little baby, you'll agree that paying attention can be easy.

The Harvard psychology graduate student Matthew Killingsworth and Professor Daniel Gilbert tracked the momentary moods of more than two thousand volunteers by creating an iPhone app that polled them at random moments. The title of their published paper tells it all: "A Wandering Mind Is an Unhappy Mind."[70] They found that respondents' minds wandered about half the time but that their moods were brightest when they were absorbed in a task. Surprisingly, positive daydreams felt just as good as but no better than being absorbed in a task. Neutral and negative mind wandering felt worse.

The connection between attention and pleasure has something to do with the brain chemical dopamine. It's released when we feel desire and flows most powerfully when we encounter novel things. As long as the dopamine is flowing, we want to keep doing what we're doing. We're absorbed. But once we get enough of something — food, for instance — we become satiated, and our dopamine level drops off. Then our attention fades, too, and the mind wanders, looking for something else to get the dopamine flowing again.[71]

Learning how to find novelty in the smallest details of daily life and becoming absorbed in them — that's what mindfulness is — produces a stream of dopamine and a continuous feeling of "Yes, yes, keep doing it."

The psychologist Ellen Langer says that most people don't know the right way to pay attention; they confuse it with staring. At the talk I attended at MIT's Media Lab, she asked us to hold out a finger and pay attention to it. "Is this boring or what?" Langer asked.

"Now mindfully attend to your finger, and that means notice different things about it," she said. Her finger, she said, looked fat; it had a new red mark on it and a fingernail that needed tending. "You should feel the difference. Attending mindfully is easy.

"Mindfulness is energy begetting, not consuming," Langer added. "It's the way you are when you're at leisure, when you're traveling."

If mindfulness produces a sense of freshness and novelty, why is it so hard to pay attention? Langer said she's asked students and teachers what it meant to pay attention. "They all say, 'Hold the image still as if you're looking through a camera,'" Langer said, adding, "It's the wrong instruction."

Staring leads to boredom. Paying mindful attention means looking at the same old thing in new ways: examining overlooked details or considering it from a different angle. William James conveyed this idea in his 1899 *Talks to Teachers*:

> Try to attend steadfastly to a dot on the paper or on the wall. You presently find that one or the other of two things has happened: either your field of vision has become blurred, so that you now see nothing distinct at all, or else you have involuntarily ceased to look at the dot in question, and are looking at something else. But, if you ask yourself successive questions about the dot, — how big it is, how far, of what shape, what shade of color, etc.; in other words, if you turn it over, if you think of it in various ways, and along with various kinds of associates, — you can keep your mind on it for a comparatively long time.[72]

Langer believes that everyday mindfulness can bring you to the sweet spot between boredom and anxiety that the psychologist Mihaly Csikszentmihalyi refers to as "flow." When we feel too stimulated, we are stressed. Without enough stimulation, we're bored. Being in flow is the Goldilocks point; we're absorbed but not overstimulated.

Csikszentmihalyi's writings on flow emphasize the feeling of being "in the zone" experienced by athletes and artists performing at their peak. Yet Csikszentmihalyi also cites a case of a man who achieved flow by closely observing the rooftops of decrepit Chicago buildings on his daily train commute. "For the trained eye, even the most mundane sights can be delightful," Csikszentmihalyi writes.[73]

It's easier to find delight in the extraordinary. However, it's not the rarity of the subject, but rather the attention which we bring to it, that produces pleasure.

This mindfulness seems like some kind of lobotomy. The capacity for thought is the highest attribute of humanity. Why should we stop thinking?

The important thing to recognize is that mindfulness is voluntary. It's a skill. It's something you can turn on and turn off when you want to. For instance, when I was a reporter covering town-hall business, I would write on deadline and file my story. Yet after the piece was completed and edited, my brain would still be working on it, suggesting belated wording changes. It's useful to be able to turn down repetitive thinking when it's no longer productive.

That being said, and I don't want to frighten you, there is a resemblance between the effects of mindfulness and aspects of Alzheimer's disease. In his 2001 book *The Forgetting*, David Shenk relates the experience of Morris Friedell, who was in the early stages of Alzheimer's: "With less of a grip on what happened two hours or ten minutes ago, Morris reported feeling dramatically more involved in the present. 'I find myself more visually sensitive,' he said. 'Everything seems richer: lines, planes, contrast. It is a wonderful compensation.... We [who have Alzheimer's disease] can appreciate clouds, leaves, flowers as we never did before.'"[74]

This sounds very much like the experience of sensory amplification that occurs on emerging from meditation. As individuals like Friedell begin to lose their memory, they appear to lose the ability to match sense data with patterns stored in memory and impose those patterns on their recent experience. Therefore, they experience what is coming from their senses more directly and with less alteration from prior memories.

This is obviously something nobody chooses as a permanent state. But to be focused on the present, to be able to quiet the inner voice when we choose, has its advantages. These abilities are tools. There is no commandment that we have to use them all the time.

If you are a highly educated individual, you probably know how to turn on your brain to focus on complex problems. But do you know how to turn it off? Mindfulness can help you find the right balance.

Is mindfulness an irresponsible philosophy of living only for today?

In his 1999 book about psychopathy, *Without Conscience*, Robert Hare writes: "Although a student of New Age philosophies might shudder at the desecration of sacred principles, much of the psychopath's behavior and motivation makes sense if we think of him or her as a person rooted completely in the present and unable to resist a good opportunity."[75] That assessment certainly does make me shudder. The ability to focus entirely on the present moment can be used for good or bad.

It's critical to combine a present-moment focus with a spirit of *metta* — benevolence or loving-kindness. Mindfulness in the Buddhist tradition and also in secular humanist practice does call for such a spirit.

And despite its present-moment focus, I haven't found that mindfulness makes you more impulsive — rather the opposite. When you are mindful, you examine everything, including your own motivations, and so it may actually make you more deliberate.

You might wonder if a person who is full of compassion and totally focused on the present may ignore questions about how they will survive and prosper in the future. The Buddha himself is said to have renounced a life as an aristocrat to become a wandering mendicant. Many of the Buddha's early followers appear to have done the same, giving away their wealth and living on alms. Only later did great monasteries with landholdings arise. The culture of ancient India supported religious mendicants, allowing a few individuals to be totally focused on the present moment with little need to plan for the future.

Of course, not everyone could live this way. As in any society except hunter-gatherers, some people needed to plan for the future, planting crops and harvesting food. But are future planning and mindfulness inherently incompatible? Buddhists teach that you can think about the future mindfully by *knowing that you are thinking about the future*. You can even add a mental comment like "planning, planning." Personally, I find that if I'm having anxious thoughts about the future, I can step back and notice that they are just thoughts. But if I'm actually trying to plan something constructively, such as the steps I need to do to accomplish a project at work, injecting this note of self-consciousness distracts me from the task.

What I do find useful and inspiring is to bring the attitude of *metta* — of kindness — to planning for the future.

Is mindfulness some kind of trance?

Mindfulness is paying attention to the present moment. The word *mindful* in everyday language means being attentive and careful. It is therefore the precise opposite of being spaced out.

It's true that when you emerge from meditation, you may be in an altered psychological state, in particular with the inner voice quieted. You may be so immersed in the present that you're not thinking ahead, not even for a few moments.

A few years ago, for instance, I left the Cambridge Insight Meditation Center feeling peaceful after practicing both sitting and walking meditation. My mind was quiet, and as I strolled home along the sidewalk, I continued to pay close attention to my footsteps. I approached a corner where there was a convenience store. A car on the intersecting street cut through the parking lot to avoid a red light and almost hit me.

I was being mindful of my feet, but not mindful of my environment. In paying attention to the present moment, you need to adjust the scope of that attention to the environment that you are in.

Does mindfulness make you too passive?

When being mindful, we take an accepting, benevolent attitude toward whatever is going on. And, given the way the brain works, when we accept what is, rather than clinging to how we want it to be, the sense of alarm we call suffering abates.[76] We can eliminate suffering by accepting everything. But in my view, accepting literally everything would make us too passive. Complete acceptance can help us eliminate our own suffering, but surely there are things we ought not to accept, even if we have to suffer to confront them: genocide, for instance.

If our goal is to reduce suffering overall and in the long term, then it may be best to reject rather than accept what is going on at present and to actually change the situation rather than change our emotional reaction to it. It may be possible to accept things emotionally while still maintaining a determination to change them, but without the goad of emotion, our determination to challenge wrongs may be attenuated.

It comes down to a matter of judgment. Which is worse, the present reality or our suffering? If the former, we should change reality. If the latter, we should accept reality and let go of our pain.

In this approach I follow the logic of the Serenity Prayer, which was composed by the American pastor Reinhold Niebuhr in 1943 and gained fame when it was adopted by Alcoholics Anonymous. Niebuhr was influenced by ancient Stoic philosophers such as Epictetus, who said, "We must make the best of those things that are in our power, and take the rest as nature gives it."[77] The formulation by Epictetus, which is not a prayer, is entirely suitable for humanists. Niebuhr's formulation has the benefit of greater clarity. It's easy to secularize, so how about this for a humanist serenity statement?

> I'd like —
> The serenity to accept the things I cannot change,
> The courage to change the things I can,
> And the wisdom to know the difference.

Many modern people have a bias toward changing society rather than accepting injustice. That's good. Not everything can be changed, however: each one of us, for instance, will eventually die. Acceptance must be part of everyone's repertoire, but it shouldn't be the only tool in our toolkit.

We're trying to get to a place where we do have preferences, but we're not strongly attached to them. When we're in this place, our internally generated sense of well-being is so strong that it's not drained by failure or swamped by success. Even though we'd like to achieve our goals, we'll be okay if we don't.

I find it difficult to relate to Eastern philosophy. Are there examples of mindfulness in American literature?

Henry David Thoreau was perhaps the first to import Eastern philosophy to American shores when his 1844 translation of *The Lotus Sutra* became the first Buddhist text to be published in the United States. In *Walden*, Thoreau makes several references to the "present moment," in the same sense that we use the expression in mindfulness practice today.[78] For example, Thoreau writes: "In any weather, at any hour of the day or night, I have been anxious to improve the nick of time, and notch it on my stick too; to stand on the meeting of two eternities, the past and future, which is precisely the present moment; to toe that line."[79]

He compares the freshness of the present moment to the blossoming of a flower: "I did not read books the first summer; I hoed beans. Nay, I often did better than this. There were times when I could not afford to sacrifice the bloom of the present moment to any work, whether of the head or hands."[80]

In this passage, Thoreau expresses a sense of friendliness and loving-kindness toward the nature around him, even those aspects conventionally seen as dreary:

> In the midst of a gentle rain while these thoughts prevailed, I was suddenly sensible of such sweet and beneficent society in Nature, in the very pattering of the drops, and in every sound and sight around my house, an infinite and unaccountable friendliness all at once like an atmosphere sustaining me, as made the fancied advantages of human neighborhood insignificant, and I have never thought of them since. Every little pine needle expanded and swelled with sympathy and befriended me. I was so distinctly made aware of the presence of something kindred to me, even in scenes which we are accustomed to call wild and dreary, and also that the nearest of blood to me and humanest was not a person nor a villager, that I thought no place could ever be strange to me again.[81]

In his 1849 book *A Week on the Concord and Merrimack Rivers*, Thoreau describes something akin to mindfulness of sound:

> Far in the night, as we were falling asleep on the bank of the Merrimack, we heard some tyro beating a drum incessantly, in preparation for a country muster, as we learned, and we thought of the line, —
> "When the drum beat at dead of night."
> We could have assured him that his beat would be answered, and the forces be mustered. Fear not, thou

drummer of the night; we too will be there. And still he
drummed on in the silence and the dark. This stray sound
from a far-off sphere came to our ears from time to time,
far, sweet, and significant, and we listened with such an
unprejudiced sense as if for the first time we heard at all.[82]

Thoreau's friend and mentor Ralph Waldo Emerson, in his
1836 essay "Nature," writes about the joy of seeing mindfully
with what could be called a Zen beginner's mind:

To speak truly, few adult persons can see nature. Most
persons do not see the sun. At least they have a very su-
perficial seeing. The sun illuminates only the eye of the
man, but shines into the eye and the heart of the child. The
lover of nature is he whose inward and outward senses
are still truly adjusted to each other; who has retained the
spirit of infancy even into the era of manhood.... Crossing a bare common, in snow puddles, at twilight, under a
clouded sky, without having in my thoughts any occur-
rence of special good fortune, I have enjoyed a perfect
exhilaration. I am glad to the brink of fear. In the woods
too, a man casts off his years, as the snake his slough,
and at what period soever of life, is always a child. In the
woods, is perpetual youth.[83]

Are there precedents for mindfulness in earlier periods of Western culture?

There are striking similarities between Buddhism and the ancient
Greco-Roman philosophy of Stoicism. Both emphasize that our
minds can control our feelings and that our happiness is not determined by external circumstance. Both see negative judgments as a
source of suffering. Both emphasize being in the present moment.
In his *Meditations*, the Roman emperor and Stoic philosopher

Marcus Aurelius writes, "Man lives only in the present, in this fleeting instant: all the rest of his life is either past and gone, or not yet revealed."[84]

The Stoic philosopher Epictetus said that it's not external circumstances, but our judgments about them that lead to suffering: "What disturbs men's minds is not events but their judgments on events. For instance, death is nothing dreadful, or else Socrates would have thought it so. No, the only dreadful thing about it is men's judgment that it is dreadful. And so when we are hindered or disturbed or distressed, let us never lay the blame on others but on ourselves, that is, on our own judgments."[85]

Marcus Aurelius also writes something in the *Meditations* that's a little difficult to parse but basically says that the only thing you really have control over is your own mind in the present moment: "To the mind, the only things not indifferent are its own activities, and these are all under its control. Even with them, moreover, its sole concern is with those of the present moment; once they are past, or when they lie still in the future, they themselves at once come to be indifferent."[86]

The close resemblance of Stoic and Buddhist ideas could be a coincidence, but more likely stems from early cultural contact between Greece and India.

The historical Buddha, Siddhartha Gautama, died in India around the time Socrates was born. According to Stephen Batchelor, several of the Buddha's close associates were students in Taxila, an Indian city controlled by Persia that may have hosted a Greek colony. If one can believe the traditional literature, the Buddha himself knew enough about the Greeks to contrast their system of slavery with the Indian caste system.[87]

The everyday meaning of *stoicism* has shifted to the point where it now often indicates an uncomplaining disposition or a false front of serenity that conceals suffering. For instance, in his memoir about the tragic 1912 British expedition to the South Pole, Apsley Cherry-Garrard wrote, "There wasn't an officer on the ship who did not shift coal till he was sick of the sight of it, but I heard no complaints."[88] These men were suffering but simply kept their mouths shut. (Ironically, Cherry-Garrard's book is entitled *The Worst Journey in the World*, so perhaps he was not above a wee bit of complaining.) This is not the Stoicism of Epictetus or Marcus Aurelius, which emphasized changing one's inner feelings, not simply concealing them.

PART THREE

Cultivating Joy

CHAPTER THIRTEEN

Walking Meditation

TYPICALLY, PEOPLE THINK OF MEDITATION as something you do while you're sitting down. But you can actually meditate in a number of postures, and even while you're moving. The four classic Buddhist postures for meditation are sitting, standing, lying down, and walking. A standing meditation is often recommended as an antidote to drowsiness. If you're nodding off during a sitting meditation, you can try standing up and see if that keeps you awake. The body scan meditation can be done while lying down. But walking meditation, too, is a form of mindfulness meditation in which you are mindful of the body and engage your sense of touch.

Walking meditation is something often done *after* a sitting meditation. If you do a daylong retreat, it's good for the muscles to alternate periods of sitting and walking.

In a formal walking meditation, you usually walk fairly slowly, but you can walk at any pace you wish.

Exercise: Walking Meditation

Allow 5 to 10 minutes for this exercise, in addition to any preceding sitting meditation. Find a place where you can both sit and walk. If you are indoors, there will probably be a chair handy, but you will also need a clear area where you can walk. If there is enough room, you can walk in a circle. With less space available, you can walk back and forth in a straight line — not tensely pacing, but in a relaxed way.

A public park is a nice place in which to do this outdoors. You will need to find a bench or a ledge on which you can sit for a few minutes. Alternatively, you can bring a blanket and sit cross-legged on the grass.

Start with a sitting meditation, such as mindfulness of breath or mindfulness of sound. Sit for as long as it takes to settle your mind. Then get up and walk!

As you walk, focus on the soles of your feet as they contact the floor or earth. You can also pay attention to the movements of each leg as you lift it, move the leg forward, and place your foot down.

Sometimes I find it useful to pay attention to the entire leg below the knee. If you're walking fast, you can pay attention to the motion of the entire body, including the arms.

You can also make mental notes as you lift and place each foot. When lifting the foot, you might say quietly to yourself, "Lifting." When placing the foot down, you might note quietly, "Placing." Those notes are not meant to be commands to the foot to control your walking but simply observations of what has just happened. Just as trying to control your breathing can lead to anxiety, trying to control your foot placement may interfere with a meditative state. Let your feet move automatically, and note what they do. Your awareness should be slightly behind the action so that you're observing it and not controlling it.

If you are doing this indoors, walk with a lowered gaze, looking toward the floor a few feet ahead of you or, if you're in a group, at the back of the person walking in front of you.

If you're outdoors, you may feel less self-conscious if you walk at a normal pace. That way, no one will know you're doing a walking meditation. Don't restrict your attention as narrowly as you would indoors — you don't want to get run over by a car or hit by a bicyclist. Look around and listen as you walk. Stay in the present moment, but keep a wide focus.

Walking meditation can be an opportunity to practice loving-kindness. As you walk past someone, you can treat them as the neutral person in *metta* practice. Think:

I'd like you to be safe
I'd like you to be healthy
I'd like you to be happy
I'd like you to be at ease in the world

If you are walking in a circle as part of a group, you may find yourself judging others, or yourself, for walking too slow or too fast. If so, this is an opportunity to practice *metta* toward the person who seems out of step.

Discussion

One of the first times I did a walking meditation was at Henry Thoreau Zen Sangha, a Buddhist community affiliated with a Unitarian Universalist congregation in a suburb of Boston. As we circled around the sanctuary in slow motion, thoughts and images arose, among them John Cleese's "silly walks" routine from *Monty Python's Flying Circus.* You may well feel silly the first time you do walking meditation, but after a while, you get used to it.

Another time, I participated in an outdoor walking meditation led by a Buddhist monk associated with the Plum Village community of the Vietnamese Zen master Thich Nhat Hanh. The monk suggested we think of each step as if our feet were "kissing the Earth." I liked that image and found it worked for me.

When I combine *metta* practice with walking meditation, I'm tempted to smile at people or say hello. In Boston, though, saying hello to someone you pass on the street is generally not done. If you live in a place where people are reserved, it may be best to avoid the hello — but you still might get away with a smile.

Questions to Consider

Where in your body were you most attentive to the experience of walking? Was it in your feet, or did the awareness travel up your body?

Did you settle into a rhythm?

Under what circumstances, if any, would you say hello to a stranger you pass on the street?

Would you be embarrassed to be seen walking slowly in a public park?

What sort of opportunities do you have on a typical day to turn a routine stroll into a mini-walking meditation?

Laura's Story

Growing up, Laura's impression of meditation — from a distance — was that it was "pretty New Age-y ethereal, what we now call 'woo-woo.' It was somewhat negative and definitely uninformed," she said.

"Subsequently, I was introduced to what it really is, in a way, through a back door. It was through some dance classes." Her ballet teacher's instructions on how to pay attention to the body were in effect Laura's introduction to mindfulness. "It helps you to cultivate a hyperattentiveness to what's going on in your body and what is going on around you," Laura said. "She never called it that, but through the processes of floor-barre and barre exercises and the way she taught us to dance, she cultivated that sensibility."

That practice of attentiveness is useful in her professional work as a landscape designer. "My experience at the drafting board and learning how to draw, and also in starting to make art, mostly drawing and painting — I realized that it was that same mindfulness that benefited the creative processes of all those activities....I essentially meditate as I work. Meditation was never something that I learned to do in and of itself. It was always something that was informing another activity."

Laura had never meditated with a group before coming to the Humanist Mindfulness Group. Our balance of combining meditation with a skeptical, inquisitive spirit has worked for her. "Because it's a meditation group, because it's a humanist mindfulness group and a secular Buddhist group, the underlying ethic of the group is one I really like and agree with. It's very *accepting*, it's very open and at the same time very grounded in the real world."

We try to experiment with a variety of different meditations, and one that was new to Laura was loving-kindness meditation. "The *metta* meditation is one I never tried before. When I first heard of it, I was a little suspicious." She laughed. "Like I'm supposed to be sending vibes." But we're very explicit that when we cultivate loving-kindness, it happens in our brains, and only affects others if we translate our feelings into behavior. "I've really enjoyed it and I've gotten a lot out of that one," Laura said. "That's helped me and so I've begun to do that one on my own."

CHAPTER FOURTEEN

Walking in the City or Suburbs

MODERN CITIES ARE full of human-made wonders. First-time visitors to Manhattan crane their necks and gasp at the soaring skyscrapers. Cities have their pockets of grime and ugliness, too. This is where nonjudgmental acceptance of the present moment comes in. Just as we can experience "noise" as mere sounds that help us to do a sound meditation, dirt and grime can be seen simply as color and texture elements that provide us with visual stimulation. A surface of peeling paint, viewed nonjudgmentally, provides novel visual elements that a fresh, uniformly painted wall often lacks.

I do prefer places that look spiffy rather than grimy. But if I happen to be somewhere grimy, and it's not my place to clean it up, I can take in the grime mindfully, without aversion. Of course, if one is in a place that is so polluted and noxious as to be a genuine health risk, feelings of disgust and aversion are appropriate. One ought not to try to overcome them with mindful acceptance.

The suburbs present a different challenge. Rather than being overly stimulating, they often seem bland and monotonous. Here, mindfulness can help us find novelty within the familiar. Look at houses. Even if they seem cookie cutter, you'll probably notice distinctive features once you start paying close attention. Simply the way they occupy three-dimensional space occupies my interest. Flowers and shrubs can be their own little natural worlds if you look at them closely.

Exercise: Walking in the City or Suburbs

If you can, start off with ten minutes of a mindfulness of breath or other sitting meditation.

Now, go outside into the city or suburban environment. Look around. Does the world look like a 3D movie that you find yourself inside, or is it a bit flattened, as in a painting? Do objects pop out of the scene, or does everything seem to lie flat? Even though the world exists in three dimensions, we often don't notice depth unless we pay attention to it.

If it feels comfortable, as you're walking, try resting the tip of your tongue on the roof of your mouth. I find that this quiets my inner voice. As a result, objects like trees, hedges, and even mailboxes seem to pop out in space, giving them a fully three-dimensional appearance.

Don't become so absorbed in any one thing that you fail to look where you're going. Whenever you come to a street or driveway, watch for moving vehicles.

Everyday Adventure

In a letter he wrote on visiting Italy in 1786, the German dramatist Goethe observed, "One agreeable aspect of travel is that even ordinary incidents, because they are novel and unexpected, have a touch of adventure about them."[89]

With mindfulness, you can find the novel and unexpected

wherever you are. The former *New Yorker* writer Tony Hiss kicks off his book *In Motion: The Experience of Travel* by relating the adventure of mailing some bills in his own neighborhood:

> Before the door had even closed behind me, the familiar world outside immediately seemed unexplored. That comes closest to describing the unexpected sensation that had arrived. "Fresh" and "new" were part of it, but only a part, even though there were undoubtedly now some things present that hadn't ever previously appeared on my block, such as the particular play of light on the buildings across the street, and the array of zigzaggy clouds in the sky overhead, and the patterns formed by the various groups of people walking by.[90]

Hiss goes on to describe how an old, battered, blue corner mailbox he'd seen many times before, in his attentive mental state, became an object of fascination. When I'm fully mindful, I experience the urban environment in the same way, with a heightened interest in shapes, light, and shadow, and even the choreography of pedestrians on their way to work. And no, I'm not on drugs — except whatever my brain produces when it's in a mindful state.

CHAPTER FIFTEEN

Mindfulness in Nature

IT'S EASY TO PAY ATTENTION when you're standing before a panorama of great beauty — the Grand Canyon, the Matterhorn, the Pacific Ocean. With so much to look at, these vast sights and the intricacies of their shapes thrill us and force us to take notice. But perhaps even a love of natural wonders needs some cultivation. I know more than one young person who has found Yellowstone National Park boring. In the United States, the number of national park visits per person peaked in 1988. The subsequent decline has been attributed to the rise of video games, home entertainment systems, and the internet.[91]

Cultivating a keen sense of observation pays dividends not only in scenic locations but also close to home. A nature walk a few years ago was a real breakthrough for me. I had just driven out to central Massachusetts to have lunch with a friend and was returning home. To keep myself entertained, I'd been listening to a tape in the car. I had some extra time, so I decided to take a detour to Hopkinton State Park, which has a reservoir created by a dam. Here is my journal entry for that day:

> Walking across the dam, I paid attention to my steps, as
> in a walking meditation. It didn't click in at the dam, but

when I got to the other side with the trails and a bird making woodpeckerish sounds, a meditative mind clicked in.
Walking back across the dam, I was aware of individual
tufts of grass. My meditative mind stayed with me driving home. I did not listen to the tape. It's still with me
now, six hours later. I've done some computer work and
watched TV, but by mental noting, I think I've kept in
touch with it. It was in the *Four Foundations of Mindfulness* book, to do constant mental noting. The mind isn't
perfectly quiet, but the inner voice volume is low — but
not so mute that I can't think ahead to dangers while driving, but perhaps quiet enough not to ruminate.

The book *The Four Foundations of Mindfulness*, by U Silananda, a contemporary Buddhist monk, is a commentary on the
ancient Buddhist discourse about mindfulness. What stuck in my
mind particularly was a story it relates about a monk who, in his
daily wanderings, ardently cultivated mindful walking: "When he
had gone four or five steps without mindfulness, he would go back
to the place of the first step and start to practice again."[92]

Since this breakthrough, I've had a chance to see how the sense
of wonder brought on by mindfulness compares to that brought
on by natural wonders. When my wife and I traveled to Ireland,
we visited the Cliffs of Moher, with a seven-hundred-foot sheer
drop into the waters of the Atlantic. They were stunning. They
riveted my attention — at first. We walked along the clifftops,
exploring new vistas. On the way back, though, the scenery was
familiar, and my attention drifted. I caught myself and decided to
pay attention to my steps and to the grass in the pastures that run
up nearly to the cliff edge. That effort brought my sense of wonder back, and for some reason, I became particularly mindful of
sound. I felt the same sense of wonder that I'd experienced while
viewing the cliffs minutes before.

The truth is that, like all other feelings, the sense of wonder is generated within our brains. Some things, like dramatic cliffs, are better at stimulating our brains to produce the sense of wonder. But when we become skillful at mindfulness, we can produce these states in ourselves just about anywhere.

Exercise: Mindful Hiking

Pick a local hiking spot. It doesn't need to have great views or other special attractions. Mindfulness will bring out the extraordinary in an ordinary tract of woods.

Sit down on a bench, a comfortable rock, or patch of grass. Meditate on your breath, or on sound, for at least ten minutes. You might want to keep your eyes open just slightly while you meditate, so that you don't get spooked if an animal or another hiker suddenly appears.

Once you emerge from the meditation, start walking. Notice the feel of your feet as your boots touch the ground. Listen to your footsteps as they crunch on fallen leaves, to the sound of birds, and to the wind as it rustles leaves. Notice the scent of any trees or flowering plants. Notice the trunks of the trees and the way they hold up a canopy of leaves. See them in their full three-dimensionality, their full "treeness." Do the same with stalks of grass and weedy plants.

Don't forget to notice your own body and how it is situated in this environment. You are a part of nature.

To help you notice your three-dimensional or stereo vision, you might try this. Close one eye or cover it with the palm of your hand. Now, look off in a new direction, to your left, to your right, or behind you. Notice the various plants and try to guess which are closer to you. Finally, remove your hand, or open the closed eye. Did you guess right? What's different when you see with stereo vision? Did something open up? Have the spaces between the leaves changed in their appearance?

Try alternating between a narrow focus in which you concentrate on one item, such as a stone or plant, and a wide focus on the sweep of everything around you.

I used to find hiking kind of boring until I got to the top of a mountain and enjoyed the sweeping views. Walking through the woods was the boring slog necessary to reach a rewarding vista. Now, however, by practicing mindfulness while hiking, I find the formerly boring flat woodlands just as rewarding as the view from the top.

CHAPTER SIXTEEN

Mindful Manual Labor

WASHING THE DISHES. What drudgery! But bringing mindfulness to almost any manual task can make it more enjoyable: raking leaves, gardening, housework.

Part of the reason we get bored is that we cut ourselves off from the sensations around us. If we can do a task without paying a lot of attention, we think we're better off if we don't pay attention. But if we do pay close attention, there can be a lushness to the sensations. It's worth a try.

Exercise: Mindful Washing of Dishes

The meal is over. There are dishes in the sink.

Before tackling the dishes, take five minutes to sit and bring your mind to stillness. Loosen any tightness in your jaw, tongue, and lips.

Now, start on the dishes.

If you scrape food off the dishes, what sounds do you hear? Perhaps there's a whoosh as you turn on the faucet. Feel the temperature of the water on your fingers, the slipperiness of the soap, and perhaps how light reflects on the dishes.

Notice the weight of the dish in your hand. Be inside your hands and notice the movements of your muscles as you rub the dish clean.

Kieran's Story

Before moving recently, Kieran taught English as a second language in the Boston area. He has also been forging his own path combining Buddhism and Hindu philosophy in a secular context.

Kieran was first exposed to Eastern philosophy in high school. At Sarah Lawrence College, he attended a talk by Stephen Batchelor, a former Buddhist monk who is one of the leading voices in secular Buddhism. Batchelor cofounded a program in Buddhist Studies at Sharpham College in the United Kingdom, which Kieran attended as part of his junior year abroad.

"It was delicious. It was quite nonacademic. Like, I don't think we had homework once the whole time there. We'd have a few classes a week. We'd also work in the garden, meditate together mornings and evenings," Kieran said. "We were in an old English country house...in the crook of this tidal river. It was an incredibly luxurious situation."

Back in the United States, Kieran became a resident at the Springwater Center in upstate New York. The center was created by Toni Packer, who was trained in Zen and selected by the teacher and author Philip Kapleau as his successor at the Rochester Zen Center. Instead, she broke away from the Zen tradition to create a less structured program.

"She started this place that experimented in a very intelligent way with what was worth keeping in Zen forms and what wasn't particularly conducive to people deepening their inquiry. Among other things there was quite an emphasis on nontechnical meditation," Kieran said. "Just being with your experience moment to moment, open listening, receptivity."

Kieran refers to this as "choiceless awareness" or "nonmeditation" and says that striving too much to be a good meditator can actually be a block to success. "I've seen many people who have practiced effortful techniques for years and years and years, and there is a way that they've never noticed an ever-present possibility that is there from the very first time they sit down. It doesn't require concentrative skill."

Kieran joined the staff at Springwater and was there for seven years, but eventually, he grew curious whether his meditation practice could survive contact with the outside world. He came to Boston and began teaching.

"In certain ways my contemplative life flowered as it hadn't before," Kieran said. "For one thing, this subtle division between formal meditation practice and daily life was eroded further. As I swagger about my day, meditation is very available."

CHAPTER SEVENTEEN

Mental Noting of Actions

HAVING A QUIET MIND IS LOVELY, and there are some simple manual tasks that you can do with a quiet mind: washing dishes, raking leaves, sweeping floors. But there are other tasks that are a bit more complex, where keeping a perfectly quiet mind may be inappropriate or even unsafe. For instance, imagine you are driving a car, and a ball rolls out into the street. If you have a perfectly quiet mind, you may be very aware of the ball — its color, its shape, and everything else about it in the present moment. But because you are anchored in the present moment, you might not think ahead to what is likely to occur in the very next moment — which is, of course, that a child might run out into the street after the ball.

It's still possible to quiet our thinking while paying attention and responding to important signals in our environment. *Mental noting*, which we encountered in the walking meditation, allows a bit of inner speech while we remain focused on the present moment.

Mental notes anchor you in the present moment and monopolize your inner speech. You come up with a word or phrase that describes what you're doing. It's like a mantra, except that the words change as you change what you're doing.

An advantage of this practice is that it can fill in the gaps be-tween the thoughts that let you keep track of what you're doing, so that distracting thoughts don't creep in. Our minds operate faster than our limbs. You can have five different thoughts while walking to the closet to find your rain jacket. By the time you get to the closet, you may have forgotten why you were going there. Mental noting keeps the focus on the present.

Exercise: Mental Noting of Actions

The first time, try this for just 30 seconds. Make a mental note of every action you do. Let's say you just arrived at your front door and are about to enter the house. Your noting might run along these lines: *reaching into pocket, pulling out key, slipping key into lock, turning knob, opening door, entering, closing door,* and *placing keys on counter.*

These are things you might do automatically, but when you note them, there is a greater intensity about them.

It's hard to do this noting for an extended period, but even a thirty-second practice will have an impact. After a while, you won't necessarily have to note your actions in words. You'll just be paying more attention to movements you otherwise do without thinking.

Next, try mental noting while you're doing something more complex, such as cooking. Assembling ingredients and preparing them in the right order takes a bit of thinking. You can't necessar-ily cook with a quiet mind, but you can focus on the task at hand by inserting mental notes. They could be *chopping, slicing, rinsing, turning on burner, covering pot,* and so on.

Notice the moments when you feel bored. What can you no-tice about the aroma, color, or temperature of the food that makes the experience more interesting? At what points are things too hectic for you to note your actions?

You may find that mental noting interferes with some activities, such as reading. Most people, including me, subvocalize as they read — pronouncing the words in their head. For me, adding the word *reading* into that inner stream of thought interferes with comprehension of the text.

While driving a car, a meditation on the breath would be unsafe, because it would take your attention away from the road. But mental noting of your driving can help focus your attention on the road. Your noting might include *checking mirror, driving, signaling lane change, checking for merging traffic,* and so on.

When you're doing this, interpret the "present moment" more broadly than you might do in a breath or sound meditation. You often need to think at least a few seconds ahead when you're driving. Think of the present as the task at hand, rather than what is happening at this exact second.

Whatever you do, remember to bring an attitude of kindness to your notes.

CHAPTER EIGHTEEN

Mindful Vision

BECAUSE VISION is the sense by which most of us, except for the visually handicapped, take in much of our information, bringing mindfulness to vision can be a great joy. But it might not be so obvious how to meditate visually. One way to see mindfully is to cultivate your attention to three-dimensional space.

Some people can't see in three dimensions. Oliver Sacks wrote an article in the *New Yorker* about such a woman, Sue Barry. She later wrote her own book, *Fixing My Gaze*. Barry was not blind, but she lacked depth perception. Although she had 20/20 vision in both eyes, they were misaligned so that she could not see in three dimensions. She could judge distances only by using other tricks, such as the knowledge that if a skyscraper looks tiny, it must be far away.

When she turned fifty, though, she finally saw a specialist who trained her to align her eyes properly. Suddenly, the world popped out into three dimensions! She was astonished. Here she writes about seeing her first snowfall with her new skill: "I could see the space between each flake, and all the flakes together produced a beautiful three-dimensional dance. In the past, the snow would have appeared to fall in a flat sheet in one plane slightly in front of me.... I watched the snow fall for several minutes, and, as I watched, I was overcome with a deep sense of joy. A snowfall can be quite beautiful — especially when you see it for the first time."[93]

People lose their sense of depth perception when under stress. When fearful, we lock onto the threat — let's say a tiger. What's behind the tiger is irrelevant. Depth perception, according to one current theory, evolved not as a defensive mechanism but rather to help our primate ancestors take advantage of opportunities for feeding, especially in trees. Under stress, the body tends to shut down functions used for feeding. As Rick Hanson, the author of *Buddha's Brain*, has quipped, before we can focus on what we'll have for lunch, we need to make sure we're not going to be someone else's lunch.[94]

By relieving stress, mindfulness can broaden your sensory focus. When this happens, the three-dimensionality of the world may seem to pop out, an effect that makes nature seem even more beautiful. I seem to be especially drawn to objects that project into space with nothing underneath them — tree branches, say, or flowers that seem too large for their stems to support. But you can experience this awareness indoors too. In a mindful state, I'm aware of how the furniture in my room and knickknacks exist in space. Even the way my laptop's power cord curls in space holds interest.

When you're in a calm, meditative state, the muscles that control your eyes relax, and the focus of your vision softens. This soft focus is the opposite of a hard, intense stare. When you concentrate on one spot, everything else goes out of focus. When you soften your gaze, you may not see that one spot quite as sharply, but you may see everything else quite a bit better.

Another reason the visual world seems more engaging when we're mindful is that we become conscious of more *novel* visual information. The brain processes a lot of visual information before we ever become conscious of it. We normally see objects as having the same color even when lighting conditions change; this phenomenon of perception is called *color constancy*.[95] Artists, on the other hand, are trained to notice color differences caused by changing light. Claude Monet painted Rouen Cathedral more than thirty times under different light.

Sometimes we take in something quickly, make an assessment, and shift our attention. When we're mindful, we hold things in our attention longer and notice overlooked elements that may turn out to be quite rewarding.

Exercise: Mindful Seeing

Allow 25 minutes for this exercise. Select a three-dimensional object that you can place in front of you. An object that is basically two-dimensional, such as a painting, is not a good choice for this exercise. I like to do this with a houseplant, or if I have them, fresh flowers in a vase. You could choose a sculpture, but you might want to choose one that generates interest because of its shape rather than one associated with a cultural or religious narrative.

If you are meditating in a group and can arrange the seating in a circle, place the object in the center of the circle.

Now, get comfortable on a cushion or chair, and do a twenty-minute meditation of your choice. It could be a breath or sound meditation, or whatever gets you into a meditative state of mind. Do this meditation with your eyes closed.

After twenty minutes, open your eyes and gaze on the plant or object in front of you. Bring the same focus and concentration to this as when you were meditating with your eyes closed. But don't stare in a single spot: move your gaze over, around, and through the object. Try to see it as a three-dimensional object in space. Notice the "negative space." If the object is a plant, for instance, notice the empty space between the leaves. Notice the gap between the plant and the potted soil.

Examine the object mindfully for at least five minutes. Notice any emotions you may feel as you do this.

Discussion

Our group first tried this practice during the December holiday season, when there happened to be a red poinsettia available. I placed it in the center of the circle. People's reactions varied depending on the angle from which they observed the flowers. One fellow said he actually found the poinsettia kind of threatening. From his angle, one pointy leaf looked like a sharp spike aimed at him. From my point of view, I found the leaves to be luxuriantly beautiful.

I haven't come across a Buddhist practice in which one contemplates three-dimensional space in exactly this way. But I have heard Buddhist teachers talking of a sense of spaciousness one experiences when mindful. I've always interpreted this to mean that part of being mindful is noticing the physical space around us and how things lie within it.

In his book *Beyond Religion*, the Dalai Lama describes a practice in which one contemplates an object such as a flower, sculpture, or painting. However, that is only the first step in the practice. The next step is to hold a mental image of the object in the mind's eye.[96] We tried this meditation in the Humanist Mindfulness Group. It was quite difficult and not at all relaxing. Even now, if I close my eyes, I can see the image of the Snoopy PEZ dispenser that I made the object of this meditation. I even see it from the specific angle from which I gazed on it as I engraved it into my memory, a view from above that emphasized Snoopy's forehead. I can imagine this technique being used to enhance one's devotion to a sacred object. In a secular context, contemplating a natural object could perhaps enhance one's commitment to conservation.

Recently, I came across a book called *The Open-Focus Brain* by Les Fehmi, a psychologist, and coauthor Jim Robbins.[97] Fehmi presents an exercise in which readers are asked to contemplate the empty space between objects. This is similar to what I'd come up with on my own, except that Fehmi expands these instructions to include an awareness not only of what is at the center of your vision but also of what is in your peripheral vision.

Fehmi argues that becoming more aware of three-dimensional space can lower your stress level. When under stress, we focus very narrowly on a threat and generally don't pay attention to visual depth. The brain has a lot of feedback loops, so it seems plausible that the process could work in the other direction and that cultivating a sense of spacious, three-dimensional vision may relax us and reduce stress. I certainly find that it brings me joy.

Questions to Consider

Were you able to be mindful of empty space?
Did you notice shadows? Textures?
Did noticing parts of an object aid in the appreciation of the whole?
How often are you aware of the space around you?
How observant are you of changes in your surroundings?
Do you enjoy people watching?

CHAPTER NINETEEN

What If You Never Saw It Again?

SOME OF THE BEST ADVICE on how to be mindful — though she never used that word — can be found in the writing of Rachel Carson, who is considered to be the founder of the modern environmental movement. In *The Sense of Wonder*, Carson writes: "Exploring nature with your child is largely a matter of becoming receptive to what lies all around you. It is learning again to use your eyes, ears, nostrils, and finger tips, opening up the disused channels of sensory impression. For most of us, knowledge of our world comes largely through sight, yet we look about with such unseeing eyes that we are partially blind. One way to open your eyes to unnoticed beauty is to ask yourself, 'What if I had never seen this before? What if I knew I would never see it again?' "[98] This exquisite way of sensing the world is what mindfulness is all about.

If you've already seen something, it is hard to imagine seeing it again for the first time (unless you do something unusual, like looking at it upside down). But you can imagine that you are seeing it for the last time, because sometimes that's true. And you can also imagine what things would be like if you'd never encountered it in the first place.

This effect has become known in the psychological literature as the George Bailey effect. It's named after the lead character in the movie *It's a Wonderful Life*, who at first is focused on all that's gone wrong in his life. Then he has a hallucinatory experience in which he loses everything he loves. When he wakes up from this nightmare, he's much more appreciative of the good things he has and less focused on what he lacks. Going through a process of imagining that positive events never happened, and then appreciating the fact that they actually did happen, has been shown in one study to improve mood.[99]

Exercise: What If You Never Saw It Again?

Imagine your house is threatened with destruction by an impending hurricane, flood, or wildfire. You've been ordered to leave your home within fifteen minutes. You may never see it again.

Go to a room in your home and try to notice everything about it, so that the memory of it will be with you always. Notice the objects in the room as well as decorative flourishes on the ceiling and window frames. If you see dust, cracks, and stains, they are just more interesting details to notice. Take it all in with nonjudgmental, loving attention.

What do you see that you haven't noticed for a long time? Do you see anything that you never noticed before?

Perhaps you'll notice some nice objects that you haven't been paying attention to lately (such as knickknacks or framed pictures). Mindfulness can freshen things up, similar to what happens when you switch knickknacks to different locations. Objects get our attention more when they're in unfamiliar contexts. With mindfulness, we can have a fresh experience without having to physically rearrange the room.

CHAPTER TWENTY

Contemplative Photography

FINDING UNUSUAL BEAUTY in everyday photographic subjects is a form of mindful seeing. We picked a lovely summer day for a contemplative photography outing. First, we walked over to John F. Kennedy Park along the Charles River in Cambridge. We were fortunate enough to find unoccupied park benches, where we sat down and meditated for fifteen minutes. No passersby paid any attention to us.

Then we got up and started taking photos. I felt a stillness in my own mind that helped me see a number of subjects as still lifes. We photographed flowers, trees, cobblestones, and buildings. Afterward, we shared some of our best photos online.

One of our photographers got down on the ground to take a wonderful close-up of a yellow flower. A passerby asked her if she was visiting from another country and had never seen a dandelion before! Mindful seeing is acting as if you really haven't seen a dandelion before.

Exercise: Contemplative Photography

Start with a silent meditation, for as long as it takes to still your mind.

Then start taking photos.

Look for small subjects, things you might walk by at other times without paying them any attention.

Look at objects that are conventionally thought to be ugly, like utility poles or manhole covers. Can you compose a shot that finds some beauty in them?

Notice your emotions, including perhaps a craving to get the next good shot. Sometimes, wanting to take a photo can get in the way of directly experiencing what is present. So don't just take the photo: give the object more time and more attention after you've taken the photo, without holding the camera between you and it.

CHAPTER TWENTY-ONE

Mindful Viewing of Museum Exhibits

PRACTICING MINDFULNESS in daily life can make the ordinary seem special. Practicing mindfulness in the presence of works of art or nature that are already special can bring our experience of them to a higher level.

Once in a while, we in the Humanist Mindfulness Group go on a field trip in order to practice mindfulness. We've visited the Harvard art museums and mindfully examined Buddhist sculptures and paintings by Mark Rothko.

When we visited the Harvard Natural History Museum, the idea was not to hurry in order to see everything but rather to pick a few exhibits and spend time with them. We started off with ten minutes of sitting meditation in the museum lobby. We then went up to the mineral and gem room, which was a visual feast. One exhibit was a 1,600-pound geode containing purple amethysts. We viewed the objects in silence and compared notes afterward.

I expected people to be mindful of the rock's visual appearance. To my surprise, participants also reported noticing the rising of thoughts and attempts to build narratives about how the rocks came to the museum. People found themselves asking questions like: Who were the collectors? What must they have felt when they came across this extraordinary sample?

Later we moved into a hall that displayed biological samples, including a human skeleton. Here we became mindful of emotions, including aversion and even fear when observing the skull's lifeless eye sockets. Nearby were birds and bats displayed not in lifelike poses, but flat and dead-looking. The corpses of beautiful kingfisher birds inspired me to feel compassion, but not those of bats. Displays of other birds in lifelike poses inspired admiration.

Later, I learned of a study by Linda Henkel of Fairfield University that looked at the impact of picture taking during museum visits. Undergraduates were asked to visit a museum and either take photos of objects or simply observe them. They were tested the next day about the objects they'd seen. Those who had taken photos had poorer recall of what they'd seen.[100] Obviously, the photo takers were not taking photographs in the same way we did in the contemplative photography exercise. When you see something amazing, there is a temptation to take the photo of it and then think you've captured the experience, without spending enough time actually looking at it.

Exercise: Mindful Viewing of Museum Exhibits

Pick a gallery, museum, or historic site to visit mindfully. A small museum with a modest entrance fee (or none) is probably better than a big, comprehensive museum like the Metropolitan Museum of Art in New York, because you don't want to feel that you need to get your money's worth and see as many objects as you can.

Before viewing the objects in the collection, see if you can find a bench and sit meditatively for five or ten minutes.

Now, get up and start to look around.

What do you see?

For the most part, don't read the descriptions explaining what each piece is. Just look at the piece.

What emotions does it inspire?

If you find a piece that is particularly striking, spend a couple of minutes looking at it from all angles. If there is a bench nearby, sit down and observe it from the bench.

Another thing you can do, especially for a large object, is to take a "mental photograph." Instead of just looking at the object as a whole, examine its constituent parts closely. See how the parts are positioned relative to each other in space. Then close your eyes and see if you can reconstruct the object in your mind's eye. The first time you do it, it's likely you will have missed some things. But if you keep opening your eyes to observe, and then closing them and trying to reconstruct the object, it's likely you will retain more than you initially thought possible.

Mindfulness and the Creative Arts

Many artists are gifted with or have learned a mindful way of seeing. In her book *Drawing on the Right Side of the Brain*, the art teacher Betty Edwards provides an exercise in which students are asked to copy an upside-down portrait of the composer Igor Stravinsky.[101] It's easier to make accurate copies from upside-down originals because when viewing an image upside down, we observe the lines and shadows as they actually are. When we view something from a familiar vantage point, in contrast, our habitual expectation of what it *should* look like influences how we portray it. We might, for instance, draw a swimming pool as a rectangle, failing to notice that its far end appears narrower due to perspective. When you undo stereotypes, and actually take a good look at the world, it's a lot more interesting.

In literature, this technique has been called *defamiliarization*. The critic Viktor Shklovsky wrote, "Tolstoy makes the familiar seem strange by not naming the familiar object. He describes an object as if he were seeing it for the first time, an event as if it were happening for the first time."[102]

The reader sees it from a new perspective unfiltered by preconceived notions.

CHAPTER TWENTY-TWO

Mindful Couch Potato

ALTHOUGH TELEVISION is often described as *mindless* entertainment, you can watch TV mindfully — perhaps not a sitcom, but definitely a performance that involves choreographed movement.

Even though I enjoyed playing soccer as a kid, like many Americans, I have found watching soccer on TV to be boring because there isn't enough scoring. Then one day, while scanning channels and coming across a game of the English Premier League, I wondered what would happen if I watched the game mindfully.

I started paying close attention to the players, and not just the one with the ball. I started paying attention to their individual steps, their slightest movements along with the passing of the ball from player to player. It produced a sense of engagement that made it, well, kind of interesting. Instead of thinking, "Wake me when they score a goal," I was actually paying attention to the game. Later, some Europeans I knew told me that for them, much of the enjoyment in "football" is in observing good play, even if it does not lead to a goal.

I also had some members of the mindfulness group over to watch the Super Bowl. We watched part of the game with the sound turned off, allowing us to focus on the game in the present moment without the chatter of the announcers to distract us. The effect was pretty cool.

Exercise: Mindful Couch Potato

You can do this exercise while watching a performance on TV or live. The activity can be a team sport like football, an individual sport like figure skating, or a dance program like *Riverdance*. You don't need to watch a whole performance this way, but just try doing it from time to time.

For instance, if you're watching American football, for each play, pick one player to focus on, whether or not that player has the ball. As you would pay attention to every one of your own steps in a walking meditation, watch that player's every step. Watch the player's motion in detail: his stride, his hand movements, and the twist of his torso.

Notice whether your own body starts to mirror the player's motion by tensing muscles similar to those the player is using on the field. Note how your emotions shift during a play.

Keep watching even after the play is over. Avoid the quick-edit style of modern TV and hold the "shot" for longer. Watch the player's reactions after the play has concluded and he has walked back to the huddle.

Try doing this exercise with the sound on mute. The chatter of TV announcers can take you out of the present moment and prevent you from focusing only on what you see.

In a dance performance, try paying close attention to a member of the corps or chorus line rather than a solo performer.

CHAPTER TWENTY-THREE

Mindful Eating

MINDFULNESS CAN BE APPLIED to all of the senses. We've already explored mindfulness of our sense of touch through both the body scan and the mindfulness of breath meditation. We've explored mindfulness of sound and vision. When we eat mindfully, we pay attention to our senses of taste and smell.

The Mindfulness-Based Stress Reduction program includes the well-known raisin exercise, which involves eating a handful of raisins with full attention. People are often surprised to find out how enlivening this exercise can be. The opposite of mindful eating is mindless eating. This can happen when you're not paying attention to your food, and you let your automatic habits control how much you eat.

I interviewed Wendy Wood, then a psychologist at Duke University, about her study of student eating habits. Wood arranged for the campus cinema to hand out free popcorn to moviegoers. Some students got fresh popcorn, and others got two-week-old popcorn, which Wood described as resembling Styrofoam.

Those in the habit of eating popcorn gobbled it up whether it was stale or fresh. Students who didn't regularly eat popcorn at movies ate the fresh but left the stale popcorn uneaten.

"People are not responding to the taste of the popcorn or the saltiness or any of the other reasons why they might think they're eating the popcorn," Wood said of the habitual popcorn eaters. "Instead, they are responding to a habit, and they perform the habit even when the popcorn is pretty disgusting."

This may seem like pop psychology, but there is plenty of neuroscience that explains how our habit system works. Once something becomes a habit, we can do it with little or no attention. This can be a good thing, because it allows us to do more than one thing at a time and makes us more efficient.

But when you eat without paying attention — mindlessly — you miss out on the experience of enjoying your meal. You don't notice when the food tastes good or even when it's subpar.

Exercise: Mindful Eating

Pick a small food item, something that doesn't require a utensil. It could be a familiar food like raisins. Or it could be unfamiliar food — perhaps something you've picked up at a farmers' market or ethnic food store. For some reason, people like to do this exercise with chocolate.

Now imagine that you are about to taste this food for the first time. Approach it with curiosity.

Inspect it visually: note its color and shape, and whether it's dull or has a sheen.

Close your eyes now if it helps you concentrate.

Bring it up to your nose and sniff. Does it have an aroma?

Bring it up to your lips, but don't eat it yet. Notice your emotions. Is there desire? Anticipation? Frustration at not having it in your mouth yet?

Now take a bite.

Notice any sound the food makes as you bite into it.

Chew it. Notice the texture. Is it hard or soft? Rough or smooth? Yielding or tough?

Notice the taste.

How do the taste and aroma play on your tongue and mouth?

After you swallow the food, how does it sit in your stomach? Does it make you feel energized or leaden?

As you continue to eat, do your desire and interest in the food diminish? Do you get to a point when you've had enough?

Discussion

Some time ago I organized a "mindful brunch" for the Humanist Mindfulness Group at a taqueria in Harvard Square. The rule was that we could chat while the food was being prepared, but once it arrived, we would spend ten minutes in silence, focused on eating. I pulled out a timer and told people to start.

We dug in. My burrito was nice and spicy, but my focused attention elevated it into something memorable. After the ten minutes were up, a fellow diner noted with surprise that he'd not completed his meal. Rather than gobbling it up, he ate slowly and, unusually for him, left some uneaten that he took home in a doggie bag. He also reported a growing sense of fullness in his stomach as he ate and a lessening desire to keep eating. If he hadn't been eating mindfully, he would have blown past those subtle signals and kept eating until he was stuffed.

If you eat slowly and mindfully, you will eat enough to satisfy your hunger, but you just might stop yourself from overeating. That's one of the messages of the 2010 book *Savor* by the nutritionist Lilian Cheung and the Zen master Thich Nhat Hanh. A third of U.S. adults are obese, more than double the rate of thirty years ago, and this increase has been linked in part to increased consumption of fast food. In addition to concerns about the nutritional content of fast food, there is a concern that the culture of eating fast may cause people to eat more than they really need. Evidence that slower eating leads to lower calorie intake is mixed, but this practice is certainly worth a try.[103]

Of course, appreciating food can be taken too far. Some people use food as a sort of therapy. A woman who indulges in ice cream as a substitute for romance has become something of a movie cliché. In one of the Bridget Jones movies, for instance, the heroine notes: "Am enjoying a relationship with two men simultaneously. The first is called Ben, the other, Jerry. Number of current boyfriends: zero." Men in movies typically find solace in beer rather than ice cream.[104] I humbly suggest that mindfulness and self-compassion practices may be a healthier way of dealing with emotional reverses.

Questions to Consider

Did you notice precisely where in your mouth taste sensations arose?

Did you notice changes to your appetite or sense of fullness during this practice?

How often do you pay full attention to your food?

Do you note cravings for particular foods?

Can enjoying just a little bit of that food satisfy your craving?

CHAPTER TWENTY-FOUR

Frequently Asked Questions about Cultivating Joy

Are the practices of mindfulness and loving-kindness just new forms of positive thinking?

They're more like positive feeling. These practices won't necessarily change the external world — just your reaction to it.

Although some scholarly research finds benefits to an optimistic attitude, other writers argue that unrealistic optimism can lead to catastrophic failures. In her book *Bright-Sided: How the Relentless Promotion of Positive Thinking Has Undermined America*, Barbara Ehrenreich takes issue with untoward optimism, blaming it for fiascos such as the real-estate bubble of the early 2000s that burst in 2008 and plunged the world into recession.[105]

The practices of mindfulness and loving-kindness are *not* aimed at controlling events in the outer world. They teach you how to tailor your inner reactions to events, to reduce your suffering, and to increase your joy. These *are* within your control.

Is mindfulness the key to happiness?

I think practices such as mindfulness and loving-kindness provide half of the key, and that is pretty valuable in and of itself.

Daniel Kahneman is a psychologist who won the Nobel Memorial prize in Economics for his contributions to the psychology of economic decision making. In a 2010 paper, Kahneman and the economist Angus Deaton asked the question, "Does money buy happiness?" They concluded that it was impossible to answer the question without distinguishing two factors that make up happiness: emotional well-being and life satisfaction.[106]

When I attended a talk by Kahneman, I asked him about these two factors. He described emotional well-being as corresponding to ongoing experience from moment to moment. By contrast, "Life satisfaction is much more of a judgment," he said. "This is what happens to you when you think about your life. You don't think about your life all the time."

Clearly, mindfulness can affect moment-to-moment emotional well-being. Intriguingly, Kahneman and Deaton found that once a household had an income above $75,000, further income made absolutely no difference in people's emotional well-being. It seems to me that, once your basic needs for food, shelter, clothing, and health care have been met, mindfulness can be the secret to moment-to-moment emotional satisfaction. It provides a tool to shift negative emotions into neutral and shift the neutral toward the positive. So that's half the secret to happiness right there.

But is a life full of moment-to-moment satisfactions a fulfilling life? Paying attention exclusively to the present moment does *not* solve the problem of long-term life satisfaction. That depends on having an overall goal or meaning to your life.

The research psychologist Roy Baumeister and colleagues have found that people often deliberately sacrifice moment-to-moment satisfaction for a greater sense of meaning, which Baumeister says involves an integration of past, present, and future states. They describe parenthood as an example of an activity that makes people less happy on a moment-to-moment basis yet is pursued because it provides a sense of long-term meaning. Political activism is another example.[107] Without a sense of direction, people can still enjoy moment-to-moment pleasures, but they lack the satisfaction of working toward long-term goals.

Although I'm not inclined toward materialistic goals, the data suggests that some people do find real long-term satisfaction by achieving them. Although Kahneman and Deaton found that additional income above the $75,000 threshold did not improve emotional well-being, it did buy more life satisfaction. In American culture, having a lot of money may not make you *feel* better, but apparently it makes you *think* more highly of yourself.

Winning the rat race does have its rewards. But when your life satisfaction depends on comparing your success to that of others, it creates a situation where some people must fall behind in order for you to get ahead.

The alternative is to search for satisfaction and meaning along a path that could be called spiritual — though humanists see that term as referring to the human spirit rather than the supernatural. It entails finding meaning through having internal goals for our character and behavior, rather than comparing our material possessions and public accomplishments to those of others.

One can even think of some Buddhist traditions as containing a career path for devotees. Mindfulness is just the beginning of the path. Although Buddhist teachings advise against becoming too attached to goals, Buddhism itself embraces the goal of progress toward enlightenment. The Buddhist devotee may also become a bodhisattva: a being who tries to help others even at the cost of deferring the experiences that lead to personal enlightenment. Combining moment-to-moment satisfaction through mindfulness with a larger goal of achieving enlightenment may provide a robust path to happiness.

Finding meaning involves thinking about the past and future, not just the present moment, so it is in tension with the present-moment focus of mindfulness. That's why I believe the attitude that comes with mindfulness — a sense of kindness or *metta* — is more important than an exclusive focus on the present. When we think about the past or future, we can do it with kindness.

How can mindfulness produce a sense of wonder?

When people emerge from meditation, they often report that sights appear more vivid and sounds more crisp. The psychiatrist Daniel Siegel, author of the book *The Mindful Brain*, suggests that this perception is the result of a competition between what he calls "bottom-up" and "top-down" flows of nerve signals inside the brain.[108]

For instance, the "bottom-up" flow associated with vision starts when light passes through the lens of the eye and falls on the retina. The retina then sends signals up the optic nerve to the brain that contain raw information about color and light intensity. To recognize that a splotch of red is actually an apple, however, the brain has to scan our memory to find a pattern that matches. This flow of remembered patterns is the "top-down" flow. The two flows come together in the cerebral cortex, where a match is made. It all happens so quickly that we're usually not aware of it. But that's how we recognize that a red splotch is an apple rather than, say, a tomato.

In fact, if the top-down patterns are unavailable, it's hard to make sense of the world. In his 1979 book, *The Brain*, Richard Restak tells the story of a man who was blinded when he was ten months old and whose sight was restored as an adult. Even though his vision was now perfect, he had difficulty recognizing objects such as the face of his doctor. As the man described it, "I saw a dark shape with a bump sticking out and heard a voice. I felt my nose and guessed that the bump was a nose, and I knew that if this was a nose I was seeing a face."[109]

Attention affects the balance between top-down and bottom-up flows. When we pay full attention, as in the practice of mindfulness, the brain changes its filter settings to increase the flow of bottom-up signals, with the result that we perceive a lot more novel sensory information. It is this novelty that excites the brain's reward system and produces the "wow."

Siegel writes, "What before was 'just a flower' can become the one-of-a-kind flower that it actually is."[110]

I asked Siegel how the maxim to "stop and smell the roses" related to his theory. Siegel answered: "Depending on the relative dominance of each flow, you can literally not bother to even experience an awareness of the scent and just go, 'Rose. Who cares? I'm late for work. Let me go,' or you can mindfully let the top-down not imprison you and spend even just five seconds with as pure a connection with the scent and sights of the rose or the thing that's in front of you as possible."

It's easier to get this sense of wonder when interacting with nature. The University of Michigan psychologists Rachel Kaplan and Stephen Kaplan have studied the restorative effects of being in nature. They theorize that because of its inherent variety and novelty, nature grabs our attention and promotes the bottom-up flow of sensations.[111]

With practice, cultivating this bottom-up flow can be done even in a built environment. When we pay close attention, the world can become a wonderland.

PART FOUR

Additional
Practices

CHAPTER TWENTY-FIVE

Mental Noting of Emotions

IN MANY OF THE PREVIOUS MEDITATIONS, we've been paying mindful attention to the world around us. In a mindfulness of emotions meditation, we turn mindfulness inward and pay attention to our feelings. This form of meditation is based on a technique I learned at a workshop led by Jack Kornfield, who encountered the Theravada school of Buddhism as a Peace Corps volunteer in Thailand in the 1960s.

In this meditation, we check in with our emotions from time to time and "note" them. We do this by coming up with a word that sums up how we're feeling at that particular moment.

When you pay attention to your emotions, you may find that they change. Usually, this attention moderates the emotion and shifts your feelings toward neutrality, particularly if the emotion is negative. If you're feeling down, and you realize, "Hey, I am kind of down," the very act of noticing seems to take the edge off despondency.

You might imagine that becoming more conscious of emotions would make them worse. But that depends on the attitude you bring to them. If you bring the attitude of aversion, you do make them worse. If you bring an attitude of kindness, you can shift them in a positive direction.

There's something paradoxical about how we deal with what goes on inside our head. It's our natural instinct to avoid unpleasant things. If you're crossing a street and a car comes speeding toward you, it makes sense to feel fear and jump out of its way. But when the unpleasant thing is inside your own brain, that strategy doesn't work well. When you have a negative feeling, and you try to negate it, you just compound it. It's not like the English language, where a double negative can be a positive. In the brain, trying to negate a negative makes things more negative.

That's because we have a conflict detector in our brain, often called the "salience network." This network of brain regions compares our present condition to our goals.[112] If what's happening at present conflicts with our goals, we start to feel alarmed. This can motivate us to avoid a negative outcome. But if the goal is related to an inner state, our instincts may work at cross-purposes with our intentions.

Imagine that you're feeling negative and want to feel happy. If you note that your inner state is negative in the present moment, and you note it *sourly*, that means you're generating another negative state to observe in the next moment. And in the next moment, you'll feel alarmed again because feeling negative conflicts with your goal of feeling happy. It's a vicious circle.[113]

Paradoxically, feeling friendly toward negative feelings mutes the sense of alarm. If you have a negative thought, and you think about it with kindness, that feeling of kindness is now consistent with your goal of feeling positive, so it doesn't trigger any further alarm. You may still have the original feeling of sadness, but you're not alarmed about feeling sad. You've stopped the downward spiral.

It's counterintuitive, but being kind to negative thoughts makes us feel better. You actually do get to change your emotions in the direction you'd like. The trick is to do it indirectly.

Exercise: Mindfulness of Emotions

Allow 20 minutes for this exercise. First of all, if you're concerned that heavy negative feelings that you've been repressing might come up if you are mindful of your emotions, you may want to either skip this meditation until you've become more skilled at self-compassion or do the meditation as part of a group that can provide support.

Start by choosing a silent meditation that works for you, such as a mindfulness of breath or mindfulness of sound. Don't select a *metta* meditation here, because in this exercise you're trying to become aware of your feelings rather than directly alter them.

During your selected meditation, every minute or so, survey your inner feelings.

Mentally note how you are feeling at these intervals by coming up with a word or phrase to label the feeling. The way I first learned this meditation, you silently repeat the word twice.

So it could sound like:

Anxious. Anxious.
(A minute later) Sad. Sad.
(A minute later) Hopeful. Hopeful.

After noting each feeling, let go of the note and return to your selected meditation.

You can play around with how you note the emotions. I like to insert a "Yes" into the note, to clarify that I'm accepting the emotion, not pushing it away. So I might think:

"Anxious. Yes. Anxious."
"Sad. Yes. Sadness."

Discussion

I find this meditation of great practical use in my daily life. I get caught up in negative emotions like everyone else, or perhaps even more so. Instinctively, I try to tell these emotions, "Stop it! Go away!" Accepting negativity with kindness isn't instinctive to me. But increasingly, I do remember to feel kindness toward myself when I notice negativity.

Part of the benefit, I think, comes from getting to say "Yes!" about something. When I am feeling negative, my mind is constantly thinking, "No!" My bodily feelings reflect the impact of the word *no*. But when I remember to ask myself, "Am I feeling down?" and come back with an answer of "Yes!," that *yes* changes things. *Yes* just feels different, even in answer to a negative question.

So this practice is kind of a trick, or what Buddhists like to call "skillful means." But being mindful of a negative emotion and bringing kindness to it can be a first step in a positive direction.

Does noting a positive emotion make you feel less positive? In my experience, no. Bringing kindness to an already positive state perhaps builds up the positivity further.

Some people in our group had difficulty with this meditation. They found they couldn't identify any latent emotion. In fact, they felt irritation and distress at not being able to articulate how they were feeling. So if you're irritated by this exercise, you can think, "Irritated." Or, if you can't come up with an emotion and you're okay with that, it may be that you are feeling content. If so, just think, "Content."

In this mindfulness of emotions practice, you don't *try* to change the emotion. You just observe it. And yet it changes. How is this so?

A standard research technique in psychology is to show the subjects photos of people whose emotions are visible on their faces. When we see emotional faces, we tend to mirror the emotion, and this response typically activates the amygdala, a part of the brain that becomes active in emotionally arousing situations.

In one study, the UCLA neuroscientist Matthew Lieberman used this technique and asked test subjects to apply a label to describe an emotive face while measuring activity in different areas of the brain. Some of the subjects were asked to choose between labels that reflected the face's gender — like "Samuel" or "Helen" — while others were asked to choose labels that matched the face's emotion, like "angry" or "scared." Those who were asked to choose between the emotional labels recorded less activity in the amygdala, suggesting that the act of labeling an emotion reduces its intensity. In these subjects, there was also more activity in the lateral prefrontal cortex, which has a role in modulating negative feelings.[114]

Lieberman calls this practice *affect labeling*. *Affect* — pronounced with the stress on the first syllable — is a term psychologists use to refer to the moment-to-moment experience of emotions, as opposed to *mood*, which is more commonly used to refer to prolonged emotional states. The psychiatrist Daniel Siegel has come up with a catchier phrase for popular use: "Name it to tame it."[115]

The research psychologist David Creswell of Carnegie-Mellon University has looked at this effect in the context of mindfulness. He used a measure called the Mindful Attention Awareness Scale to measure how predisposed a person is to be mindful. The score is based on the extent of a person's agreement with statements such as "I find myself listening to someone with one ear, doing something else at the same time." Creswell had subjects perform the same tasks of labeling faces by emotions or by gender. He found that people who were more disposed to be mindful had more deactivation of the amygdala than people who were less mindful.[116]

The study suggests that people who are more mindful are better at using affect labeling to mute negative emotions. This is consistent with the Buddhist belief that mindfulness training reduces one's emotional reactivity.

It appears that when we consciously acknowledge an emotion — when we "get the message" — the messenger goes away. This may be why, when you talk about your feelings to a friend, a therapist, or your diary, you feel better.

The initial studies of affect labeling involved negative imagery. Subsequently, Lieberman and his colleagues have found that affect labeling mutes positive feelings too.[117] Therefore, if you wanted to be strategic about this, you could practice mental labeling of emotions when you're in a negative mood, but not when you're happy.

Lieberman studied how affect labeling compares to a popular therapeutic technique called cognitive reappraisal. When you reappraise, you tell yourself a different story about the situation you're in to help yourself feel better about it. For instance, if you receive a rejection letter from a college, you might initially feel bad. But then you might come up with five reasons why you didn't want to go there anyway, and you feel better.

In this particular study, Lieberman and his colleagues showed test subjects disturbing pictures and asked them to use either emotional labeling or cognitive reappraisal. For instance, the cognitive-reappraisal subjects were told that if they saw a picture of a person lying in a hospital bed, they could tell themselves that the person was strong and would likely get better. Lieberman found that cognitive reappraisal was more effective than affect labeling in reducing feelings of distress. However, in other studies, the two techniques have had comparable results.[118]

These findings suggest that emotional labeling is not necessarily the best approach; other techniques can work just as well in helping us feel better in difficult situations. One of the advantages of affect labeling, though, is that it is always available. In contrast, reappraisal may necessitate spinning implausible yarns. For instance, in her book *The Pain Chronicles*, Melanie Thernstrom, a journalist who suffers from chronic pain, mentions an encounter with a man who had been blinded by an accidental shotgun blast. The man considered the accident a gift from God that saved him from a lifestyle of drinking that would have led to an even worse outcome. Thernstrom, a skeptic, wistfully wondered if she could invent a narrative that would allow her to frame her own pain in positive terms.[119]

Questions to Consider

Are you normally aware of being in a particular emotional state?

Do you notice more positive or negative emotions?

How quickly do emotions arise in you?

How quickly do emotions fade?

Did naming an emotion affect you in any way?

Did this meditation dredge up any "stuff"?

If so, can you process it with kindness?

CHAPTER TWENTY-SIX

Yes! We Have No Bananas

WE HAVE POTATOES. We have tomatoes. But no, we don't have any bananas. Scratch that. "Yes! We have no bananas," the grocer shouts, in the novelty song from the 1920s originally sung by Eddie Cantor.[120]

Attaching a simple "Yes!" to a negative outcome can be a surprisingly effective way to make it hurt less. This is not the same as denial; you are recognizing the reality of what has occurred but altering your reaction to it.

The British psychologist Daniel Nettle, in his 2005 book *Happiness: The Science behind Your Smile*, notes an interesting asymmetry between positive and negative emotions. Of the basic emotions — anger, fear, disgust, sadness, and joy — four of five are negative. It's not that the world is inherently a downer. Nettle hypothesizes that the diversity of negative emotions reflects the different ways we respond to danger. Anger makes us fight. Fear makes us flee. Sadness makes us immobile (and therefore harder for a predator to notice). Disgust nauseates us so that we vomit out poisons. Nettle writes:

> The function of each emotion programme is highly specific and totally different from the others. All the negative

emotions say, 'something bad has happened' but they disagree about what remedy to take....Joy, on the other hand says, 'something good has happened.' Its prescription for the appropriate remedy is simply 'don't change anything.' Though the sources and intensities of joy may vary, they all belong to the same spectrum. This is because there is only one way of going about not changing anything.[121]

If joy motivates you to "keep doing what you're doing," is the converse also true: that a willingness to keep doing whatever you're doing brings joy? In her 2003 book *Radical Acceptance*, the clinical psychologist and Buddhist teacher Tara Brach describes how she came to appreciate the paradox that saying yes to negativity dissolves it. Coming down with a sinus infection while at a meditation retreat, she overcame her natural aversion to feeling lousy:

I began to greet whatever arose in my awareness with a silently whispered "yes." Yes to the pain in my leg, yes to the blaming thoughts, yes to the sneezes and the irritation and the gloomy gray sky. At first my yes was mechanical, grudging and insincere, but even so, each time I said it, I could feel something relax in me. Before long, I started to play around with it....I began to offer the yes with a softer, more friendly tone. I even smiled from time to time — my whole drama started to seem silly. My body and mind grew steadily lighter and more open. Even the pressure in my sinuses began to ease up. The dark cloud of "no" was replaced by the expansive sky of a "yes" that had endless room for grouchiness and irritation. Critical comments continued to arise, and with yes they continued to pass. When my mind suggested that I was using a gimmick that wouldn't work for long, saying yes to the story allowed the thought to dissolve.[122]

I experienced something similar when I attended a free July 4 concert by the Beach Boys on the National Mall in Washington, DC, a number of years ago. The day was extremely hot. The press of people had turned the grass into a field of dirt, and my friend and I were far away from the stage. We were both bitterly disappointed by the conditions, but in a mood of dark humor, I said to my pal, "Isn't this great!" and he responded, "Yeah! This is great!" and we went back and forth like that for maybe thirty seconds. The strange thing was that after we were done, I really did feel great, and the feeling lasted for quite a while.

The simple acts of saying "Yes!" and "No!" have major impacts on the body and the way we feel. Try saying "Yes!" more, even in describing what appear to be negative outcomes.

Exercise: Yes! I Have No Bananas

During a formal meditation, as thoughts arise, we can let them go, like clouds drifting across the sky. But in daily life, when thoughts arise, sometimes we have to deal with them. When those thoughts are negative, our instinct may be to argue with them or negate them; but, paradoxically, we may feel better if we accept them. There is a Buddhist practice of chanting something called the Five Remembrances, which encourages an acceptance of illness, aging, and death. It can be a bit of a downer, but I've adapted it below, adding a bit of ironic enthusiasm.

Throughout the day, be mindful of the thoughts that flit across your consciousness. If you notice a negative judgment, try reframing it by simply putting a "Yes!" in front. For instance:

"Yes! I have a lot of work to do today."

"Yes! That didn't go the way I planned."

"Yes! I was rejected."

"Yes! I feel tired."

"Yes! My knee hurts."

"Yes! I'm getting older."

"Yes! I've lost something that I loved."

"Yes! I will die someday."

Discussion

Although I can't quite prove it, I think that moment-to-moment happiness basically comes down to saying "Yes!" at each individual moment rather than "No!" The stance of nonjudgmental acceptance that is part of mindfulness is not grudging acceptance, and perhaps not even unenthusiastic acceptance, but a real embrace of what is going on at present.

The feeling of "Yes!," the feeling of wanting something and liking it, is a product of the brain's reward system. The reward system is behind our every desire — for food, drink, sex, love, and even social prestige. In the early 1950s, at McGill University in Montreal, James Olds and Peter Milner made the first identification of a part of the brain's reward system. Trying to understand how learning reinforces behavior, they implanted electrodes into varying locations in the brains of living rats. The setup allowed a rat's brain to be stimulated from the outside by pressing a lever. The rats were taught how to press the lever, and some of them really liked to stimulate themselves. One rat stimulated itself 7,500 times in twelve hours! Olds and Milner concluded that the stimulation was rewarding to the rats, and the brain region that inspired the most self-stimulation, the septal area, became known as the brain's pleasure center.[123]

The same thing happens with humans. In the 1960s, Robert Heath implanted electrodes in living people who were undergoing surgery for various reasons (in an experiment that would no longer be permitted under contemporary ethical guidelines). These individuals engaged in the same behavior, stimulating themselves again and again.[124]

Kent Berridge, a University of Michigan psychologist whose research focuses on the nature of pleasure, questions whether those who self-stimulate in this way feel pleasure or a compulsion. He suggests that this phenomenon may really be about craving rather than pleasure. Addicts, for instance, sometimes crave drugs or cigarettes even when these no longer provide much enjoyment.

Berridge sees the reward system of being composed of separable components he calls "wanting" and "liking." *Liking* is the actual experience of enjoyment in the present moment. *Wanting* motivates us to act now to get something we expect to like at a moment in the future.

According to Berridge, the brain chemical most closely linked with wanting is dopamine. The positive sensations we experience when liking something are produced by internal opioids. Since opioids both produce pleasure and relieve pain, we can understand on a biological level what we know from experience — that pleasure can counteract pain.[125] What I take from this is that if we can trick our brains to like something, for instance by saying "Yes," this liking will be accompanied by the flow of opioids that we generate within our own bodies.

Of course there may be situations in which we witness harmful acts or even criminal acts to which we simply must say "No!" But there is a lot in this world to which we can say "Yes!"

CHAPTER TWENTY-SEVEN

Intentional Daydreaming

PAYING ATTENTION IS A KEY element of mindfulness. Meditation brings the mind to a settled state in which it can focus on what's present easily and without distractions. Buddhists contrast this with the state of mind in which our thoughts jump from one thing to another incessantly, which they sometimes refer to as "monkey mind." Being able to focus and settle down is considered a good thing.

Some scientists argue that this view overlooks the positive aspects of mind wandering. The psychologist Jerome L. Singer has long studied daydreams and even coauthored a paper titled "Ode to Positive Constructive Daydreaming."[126] Singer and colleagues distinguish between three types of mind wandering:

1. Positive constructive daydreaming, which is playful, imaginative, and creative.
2. Guilty-dysphoric daydreaming, which is anguished and obsessive.
3. Poor attentional control, which is the inability to focus on a task.

The third type seems the closest to monkey mind. We may be trying to do our homework or pay attention to something a coworker is telling us, but despite our best intentions, our mind drifts off. There seems to be little advantage to this type of distractibility, and clearly there is a role for mindfulness in helping us focus on the task at hand.

The second type generates the sort of self-condemning thoughts that produce suffering. Mindfulness practice aims to free us from these sorts of judgments. If you really have done something horrible, perhaps some self-critical reflection is called for. But more likely, these sorts of thoughts are harmful to you and probably not helpful to the people around you.

Supporters of mind wandering focus on the first item. Volitional daydreaming involves a deliberate choice to take time out from the day-to-day grind and open yourself up to new possibilities.

Is it possible to practice mindful mind wandering? Although this seems like a contradiction in terms, it may not be. Mindfulness is commonly defined as nonjudgmental attention to the present moment. Clearly, self-condemning thoughts or simple distraction are not mindful. But if you take a broad view of mindfulness, if you allow your thoughts to gently drift and you are conscious of doing so, you are paying mindful attention to your thoughts.

Exercise: Intentional Daydreaming

You may come up with some good thoughts in this practice, so feel free to have a paper and pen at your side to write them down. Writing them down will free you from the need to try to remember them, which could interfere with further daydreaming.

Start with a short period of formal meditation, say ten minutes of breath meditation, to allow your mind to settle.

Now start to think about what could possibly happen in the future. Allow your mind's eye to present you with suggestions.

. This is not the time for fantasies that are absurdly out of reach, like the speech you'll give following your acceptance of the Nobel Prize. Nor is it the place for counterfactuals — imagining your life if things had turned out differently. Rather, it is an opportunity to ask yourself, "What if...?" Consider what you could realistically aspire to if things went your way from this point on.

What new interest might you cultivate?

How might you go about meeting new people?

If you could do a different type of work, what might that be?

What places might you like to visit?

Where else might you like to live?

What limiting beliefs about yourself hold you back unnecessarily?

We Can't Banish All Desire

It is sometimes claimed that Buddhism seeks to eliminate desire. In fact, Buddhists distinguish between wholesome and unwholesome desires and claim that the latter lead to suffering. The Buddhist teacher Gil Fronsdal writes, "The Buddha did not teach that desire was the cause of suffering. In fact, he encouraged his followers to arouse ardent desire for liberation."[127] Thus, in fact, Buddhists consider the desire to advance in one's spiritual practice to be wholesome.

But desire can get out of hand. The reward system that is responsible for positive mental states also produces addictive behavior, as people try to recapture "highs" that provide them with an opioid lift. Liking something stimulates the desire for more of it. Children in a playground don't go down the slide once: they do it again and again. Adults often behave the same way. For instance, Dan Wheldon, the victor in the 2005 Indianapolis 500 automobile race, told ABC before the 2009 race, "When you do win it, it makes you even more hungry to win it again."[128]

Liking leads to more wanting by way of *learning*. The brain's reward system has its own form of memory, distinct from the memory by which we remember facts or stories. When we like something, the neurons in the reward system adjust themselves to reflect the experience. Let's say we come across a fruit that we've never tasted. We may take a small bite. If it's bitter, we spit it out. But if it's succulent and juicy, we feel delight. The connections among the neurons in the reward system adjust so that the next time we come across that fruit, we feel a pulse of excitement. That is the beginning of desire.

We can end up suffering when we want too much, but wanting too little is also problematic. If you had no desire at all, no appetite for food or for life, you'd have a hard time eating or getting out of bed in the morning.

To promote well-being, we need to *calibrate* our desires. This is not always easy to do. But if we're paying mindful attention, we're partway there.

CHAPTER TWENTY-EIGHT

Meditation on Whatever

ONE OF OUR MORE EXPERIENCED MEDITATORS, Kieran, introduced us to this meditation, which is often referred to as "choiceless awareness." At first it was hard to grasp, because it's a meditation on nothing and everything.

Most commonly in meditation, you pick an object of meditation and focus on it. In this particular meditation, there is no focus. You cultivate an open awareness of whatever is going on in the present moment.

Exercise: Choiceless Awareness

Allow 20 minutes for this exercise. Find a comfortable sitting position. Close your eyes or soften your gaze. Start with a few deep breaths. Let your eyes, tongue, jaw, and any other part of your body go soft and relaxed. After that, do nothing!

Let yourself go. Just notice what happens.

The trick is to take a passive attitude toward things. Don't pick and choose objects to focus on. The idea is to make this meditation as effortless as possible. Don't even try to do it. Just let it happen by not doing anything except noticing things. Let go of the steering wheel (don't do this meditation while driving, of course!).

You don't need to follow the breath. On the other hand, because you're sitting quietly, your breathing may be something you do notice. If the breath captures your attention, fine, but if your attention drifts off to the sound of a bird or a sensation in the body, that's fine too. Don't force yourself to return to the breath if your attention drifts.

Offer anything that catches your attention a friendly welcome.

Don't force yourself to relax. If you feel you are straining, even to relax, notice that. Paradoxically, letting go of the effort to relax may help you relax.

If thoughts arise, you don't need to bat them down. Watch them passively. Don't engage or add fuel to them by trying to debate or out-argue them. Even if some of them are accusatory, you can react with a mental shrug — a "whatever."

If you feel like you've become caught up in thoughts, it may be best to make a slight effort to shift your attention to something else: the sound of birds, your breathing, your body.

If bodily feelings arise, even unpleasant ones, notice them with kindness.

Play around with relaxing the boundaries of your body. See if you can let go of the distinction between feelings that arise on the surface of your body — say the feeling of contact between your rear end and the cushion or chair — and feelings that arise within your body — perhaps a twinge in the knee or tightness in the stomach. See them all as just sensations, neither inside nor outside your body, but simply in your world. As long as you are sitting, there should be no harm in doing this; if you get up and walk, of course, you do need to know where your foot ends and the floor begins.

Discussion

Many of us were confused when Kieran introduced this meditation to our community. We asked, How is paying attention to anything and everything different from just living your life?

In fact, choiceless awareness *is* very much like just living your life, except that it is choiceless and effortless. It's about living your life when you have nothing in particular to do.

This is not to say that you can go through your entire life practicing choiceless awareness. Obviously, sometimes you need to make choices, and sometimes you need to put in some effort. This form of awareness is one more tool in the kit.

This practice is also very useful if you have anxiety about your ability to concentrate on the breath or any other meditation object. The strain of forcing yourself to concentrate can make meditation more difficult. If you can just let it happen, you may find that concentration comes more easily. On the other hand, if you have a hard time getting into this practice, it can help to start by focusing for a few minutes on the breath or another specific object of meditation. After you feel settled, let go of your focus and just notice whatever comes up.

Christopher's Story

Christopher is the values-in-action coordinator at the Humanist Community at Harvard. His role is to translate the beliefs humanists have about helping others into concrete actions, including packing free meals for food-insecure families and arranging for volunteers to assist the homeless.

Christopher is also a longtime meditator. His upbringing was loosely Roman Catholic. In his teens he was introduced by his older brother to books about Eastern philosophy. He was fascinated.

"In my late teens, I started sitting meditation retreats, first at the Cambridge Zen Center," he said. "I had a crappy little car, and I would come in and sit two- or three-day intensives, waking up at 4:30 in the morning, practicing until ten at night — real hard-core training. I loved it. I kind of haven't stopped."

Christopher prefers long meditations. "I do sit a lot. I like sitting for longer periods of time, one or two hours at a stretch. I feel that that shifts my awareness palpably into a different mode of perceiving," he said. "It takes me a while to have the texture of that kind of mind, though I don't particularly want to privilege one texture over another, per se. That would be anti-mindfulness, you know, cultivating a preference for *this* rather than *that*, etc. But a certain workability and spaciousness of mind are nice. So I like to sit a bit longer to nourish that. It carries over into life in helpful ways."

Now, mindfulness is a constant. "I just took a sip of water and was conscious of the coolness of the water and the weight of the cup," he said. "It's part of my life, noting these very tactile immediate things — the sounds of the ventilation. When I studied with Thich Nhat Hanh, I got a lot out of his emphasis on walking meditation. It's very portable, nothing special, poetic without being heavy-handed or obnoxious. Just this."

Although initially, many people explore meditative practice to address their own suffering, the training can actually prepare you to deal with the suffering of others. "The biggest thing for me is the practice's ability to grant us space to rest with discomfort," Christopher said. "But if that stability and sense of safety isn't used to wake us up to a larger reality, then it becomes a kind of dead end or indulgence — maybe better than Xanax, so, okay, but rather limited in scope. Are we waking up or merely soothing ourselves? This is a burning question for me."

Mindfulness can also help in bringing sensitivity in our dealings with others. "What does it mean to go into other communities and try to help? There is a degree of self-reflexive awareness that I feel is necessary to do that kind of work authentically and with genuine compassion, not a kind of helper mentality," Christopher said.

In the twenty years since his first exposure to Buddhism, Christopher has trained in a wide variety of Buddhist traditions, including

Tibetan Buddhism at Gampo Abbey in Nova Scotia and Zen at Plum Village Monastery in France. He has gained much from the experience and relishes sitting, but he is less enthusiastic about some other practices.

"The chanting — not so much," he said. "Though certain Japanese Soto Zen liturgies and other ritual forms I have found do help to create a useful frame of mind, or a sensitivity to approach meditation with a delicate, touching something that sets the tone for deeper practice. But some forms just don't click with my peculiar aesthetic, I suppose."

Christopher considers himself a Buddhist and doesn't think that supernatural beliefs are a prerequisite. However, certain philosophical perspectives such as "non-self," or the view that what we call our "self" is not a permanent, enduring entity, are key. "The core of it for me is — unanimously among Buddhist philosophical schools — if you jettison the insight of interdependence and non-self, and you jettison the sense of a compassionate responsibility to each other and the world — those two elements — if they are displaced, I think it's inappropriate to maintain the term *Buddhist*."

It's actually for this reason that many of us in the Humanist Mindfulness Group do not fully embrace the Buddhist label. Compassion is a core value of humanism. Ideas about the self seem rather esoteric to us, though. We're open to exploring them but have yet to draw any conclusions. Christopher says that non-self is not something he embraces as doctrine but rather something he has concretely experienced as a long-term meditator.

This deeper path is not all rosy, however. "It's sometimes a very ugly business, and to prepare people, if they genuinely want to go in this direction, they should be made ready to embrace the ups and downs of it," Christopher said. "I have no doubt that cultivating a deep insight into non-self makes life better. But sometimes it gets a little worse before it gets better. It's such a radically different way of understanding life. How we create ground for ourselves, our notions of who we are, these don't go down without a hell of a fight. So, meditation practice inclining in the non-self direction shouldn't misrepresent itself as self-improvement. We should not approach it with rose-colored glasses, either. This is a tricky business, however, in a market-driven spiritual scene. If you don't want to step on that non-self path, meditation can still have great benefits. But if you want to go in that direction, it's best not to be too romantic about it."

CHAPTER TWENTY-NINE

Mindfulness of Thoughts

EARLIER, I DESCRIBED MINDFULNESS as paying attention to what is going on in the present moment, rather than thinking about what happened in the past or may happen in the future. I did note that if you step back and notice that you're thinking, you actually are being mindful of your thoughts. But I set that idea aside, because it introduces complexities. If you've followed most of the exercises this far, and in particular the preceding choiceless awareness exercise, you should be prepared to deal with this subtlety.

The idea is to take a passive approach to thoughts, to see them as events that you witness, not actions that you're performing. If, when your eyes are closed, you see a mental picture — say, piled-up papers on your desk at work — simply realize that you are witnessing an image in your mind's eye. If you hear inner speech, realize that you are observing sounds in what could be called your "mind's ear" — actually the brain's auditory cortex. These are events occurring in your brain right now, and so to notice them is to be mindful.

Exercise: Mindfulness of Thoughts

Allow 30 minutes for this exercise. Start with your favorite silent meditation, perhaps mindfulness of breath or mindfulness of ambient sound. Meditate for as long as it takes to achieve a quiet mind. Reserve at least five minutes to do the second step in this meditation, which is to witness the arising and passing of thoughts.

Let's say you have been focusing on your breath. Let that go. Relax your concentration. If a thought occurs, rather than returning to the breath, watch that thought.

Is it a word, phrase, or sentence?

Is it a wordless mental picture?

Is it a bodily feeling?

Is there a shift of sensory modes, such as a bodily feeling setting off inner speech?

What happens next? Does the thought trail off, or does it lead to another thought?

Try to take a passive approach and just witness the thoughts, without engaging with them.

If you do find yourself following a train of thought, you can let that go and return to your breath for a few moments. Once your mind has quieted again, let go of your focus and allow thoughts to return.

Continue this process for as long as it feels worthwhile.

Discussion

I first did this as part of an online meditation led by Mark Knickelbine of the Secular Buddhist Association. I found that after twenty-five or so minutes of meditation, my mind was quiet. So, when I let go of my anchor of the breath, thoughts didn't come rushing back in. Instead, what I heard were fragments — words or phrases but not full sentences. It seemed as if my brain was raising topics that could kick off an internal dialogue. At first, I just noticed them and let them go, returning to the breath. As time went on, I engaged with these topics more, allowing them to unfurl into complete thoughts of a sentence or two. Then I returned to the breath, and the thoughts subsided. I never got carried away — lost in thought — before the completion of the meditation.

Since then, I've been trying to apply this approach when I have a stray thought that distresses me — say something related to a career setback. At first, I imagine that the setback itself is what causes me to suffer, but then I remember it's how I think about it that actually causes me pain. When I catch myself in this way, I remember that my happiness is not dependent on external circumstances. By having compassion and *metta* for myself, I can return to a neutral or even joyful state.

When I catch a negative thought before it hurts me, it feels like I've caught an arrow in midflight. By noticing the arising of an accusatory thought, you can catch it before it turns into an elaborate and hurtful story.

Mindfulness of thoughts can be very helpful in dealing with stray thoughts that pop up spontaneously, including ruminations about the past and anxious thoughts about the future. It may not be helpful, however, to practice mindfulness of thoughts when one is engaging in deliberate, complex, task-oriented thoughts. So, for instance, when I'm writing these very words, if I interject an observation like "Thinking, thinking," it actually makes it harder for me to finish the sentence. I've tried practicing mindfulness of thoughts while writing a computer program, and it makes it harder for me to figure out what the next step of the program should be.[129] So don't take this practice to such an extreme that it interferes with your ability to think constructively.

CHAPTER THIRTY

Mindful Speech and Listening

IN THE HUMANIST MINDFULNESS GROUP, after we meditate, we have a discussion. In it, we try to adhere to a principle of compassionate speech. This is inspired by the Buddhist principle of right speech, though we don't hold strictly to the way that Buddhists do it.

The basic idea is to communicate with kindness in mind. Problematically, though, in traditional Buddhism, the principle of right speech includes avoiding speech that is divisive even if true.[130]

I don't think this principle works for political speech and journalism. The history of the last couple of centuries and the role of a free press in protecting liberty and exposing malfeasance indicate that we must sometimes report negative things about people. Political campaigns and litigation are inherently adversarial. Although we may wish everyone could get along, a certain amount of conflict may be inherent in a democratic system.

When we shift from the political to the personal, we can act differently. Instead of creating winners and losers, we can support each other. If you are trying to communicate with another person, rather than trying to demolish their arguments, another approach is called for.

Research by Roy Baumeister and colleagues shows that aggression is often triggered by threats to high self-regard. Mocking or diminishing a person is more likely to encourage defensiveness than inspire a change of heart. Common sense tells us that people are more likely to concede error when they can do so in a face-saving way. A recent study suggests that people are more willing to be corrected after first engaging in a practice that affirms their self-worth.[131]

At the Humanist Community at Harvard, we've had training in what is called nonviolent communication. This is a secular program created by the psychologist Marshall B. Rosenberg that is compatible with the goal of compassionate speech.[132]

The exercise below is a blend of practices from these sources.

Exercise: Compassionate Speech

Even when another person speaks angrily to you, you may respond with compassionate speech. So this practice does not require the other party in a dialogue to engage in compassionate speech too.

Before speaking:

1. Start with a feeling of kindness for yourself and for the other person. Wish the best for both of you.

2. Allow the other person to speak first. In general, people get more enjoyment out of telling others what they want than from listening to what others want. So if you allow the other person to speak first, that person may feel that the conversation is starting well and be encouraged to pursue dialogue.

3. Practice emotional acceptance of what the other

person is saying. That doesn't mean you have to agree with it or give up hope of changing the person's mind. But while you're listening, accept that, yes, the other person is saying their piece.

4. Note your emotional reactions and bodily feelings. Take a conscious breath when needed. If you feel as though you are under attack, offer yourself some self-compassion.

5. If you're feeling impatient or bored, briefly scan your body to notice what impatience and boredom feel like in the body. Rather than tuning out or interrupting the person, expand your attention from their words to their tone of voice and body language.

6. Speak subjectively rather than objectively. This is actually the opposite of what we are often trained to do in academic discourse and debate — to speak authoritatively and avoid the use of the word *I*. But where there are personal disputes, the differences are almost always subjective. They come out of values and feelings.

One advantage of the subjective approach is that it is often easier to get agreement. For instance, if you say, "What you did was outrageous!" the other person may not agree. But if you say, "I feel outraged by what you did," the other person is likely to acknowledge that you feel what you feel. The first approach brings up a "No!" and stops the conversation, while the second brings up a "Yes!" and keeps the dialogue going.

CHAPTER THIRTY-ONE

Exploring Don't-Know Mind

My first exposure to Buddhism was through Zen practice, but it did not take. Still, I learned one teaching at the Cambridge Zen Center that I do find valuable, called "don't-know mind."

The idea is to give up your preconceived notions of things. When you come across an object or situation, instead of giving it a label, you cultivate *befuddlement*. You ask yourself, "What is this?" and answer, "I don't know."

This kind of inquiry is also sometimes referred to as "beginner's mind." It's also related to Rachel Carson's practice of cultivating the sense of wonder by imagining you are seeing something for the first time.

Ellen Langer is a professor of psychology at Harvard who has focused on mindfulness in the Western psychological tradition as a form of attention training. In a talk at MIT, she described an experimental study that showed how being too fixed in our views can cause us to overlook opportunities. "What we did was to show the importance of conditional language, which is the best way to prevent mindlessness. People think they're in a consumer study. They're told, 'This is a cup. This is a watch. This is a dog's chew toy.' Or they're told, 'This *could be* a cup. This *could be* a watch.

This *could be* a dog's chew toy.'" Next, the experimenter feigns making a mistake on a survey form that could be fixed if only an eraser were handy. "Who would think to use that dog's chew toy as an eraser?" Langer asked. It turned out that only those who were told that it "could be" a chew toy considered the possibility that it could be something else — such as an eraser.

In Langer's view, being too settled in our views causes us to be *mindless*, the very opposite of *mindfulness*. We fail to notice relevant details. In the example above, those who were less fixed in their views were more imaginative and able to conceive of the chew toy as an eraser.

Labels are not always bad. In the practice of mental noting, for example, we do apply labels. Different strategies can be useful at different times. But even when mental noting, it's probably best to regard labels as provisional, impromptu descriptions rather than as fixed judgments.

Exercise: Don't-Know Mind

Go to a familiar location. Imagine that you are a detective, and that things are not what they seem. Perhaps there is a clue to a murder to be found. Examine every object, every spot on the wall or floor with a curious attitude.

Ask yourself, "What is this? Why is it here? Why is it placed just so?" What might it be, other than the obvious?

CHAPTER THIRTY-TWO

Meditative Reading

THE EXERCISES IN THIS BOOK are borrowed almost exclusively from Eastern practices. The contemplative practices of Judaism, Christianity, and Islam generally involve prayer or the contemplation of sacred texts, which makes them hard to secularize. Some, like the Jesus Prayer, seem to be a form of mantra meditation.

But I did find something interesting in the *Spiritual Exercises* of Ignatius Loyola, the founder of the Jesuit order. I attended a talk on the exercises at Harvard Divinity School by Roger Haight, a Jesuit theologian who has been punished by the Vatican for "grave doctrinal errors."[133]

One element of the spiritual exercises is to re-create Biblical scenes in your imagination with yourself as a witness. You don't make yourself one of the central characters but rather an observer. You imagine you are physically present in the scene and try to experience it with all five senses. We can do something similar with a secular text.

Exercise: Meditative Reading

When we read a good book, we tend to go through it fast. That's why it's called a page-turner. But, in line with meditative practice, what about reading something slowly, very slowly? What about allowing the sentences to bloom into vivid scenes that you experience not just visually, but with all five senses?

You can pick your own text. You might try a poem, such as Robert Frost's "Stopping by Woods on a Snowy Evening," Edgar Allan Poe's "The Raven," or Mary Oliver's "The Journey." But consider doing it with prose as well.

Here's a passage from Henry David Thoreau's *A Week on the Concord and Merrimack Rivers*, which describes a canoe trip that Thoreau took with a companion. I read this passage aloud for the mindfulness group, reading each sentence slowly. It turned out that pauses between sentences were not frequent enough to allow the meaning to sink in, because Thoreau writes in complex sentences. Below, I break up the passage into sentence fragments that each present an individual perception.

Imagine you are Thoreau's companion on this trip. Pause after each sentence fragment to let it unfold in your imagination.

Soon the village of Nashua was out of sight,
and the woods were gained again,
and we rowed slowly on before sunset,
looking for a solitary place in which to spend the night.
A few evening clouds began to be reflected in the water
and the surface was dimpled only here and there
by a muskrat crossing the stream.
We camped at length near Penichook Brook,
on the confines of what is now Nashville,
by a deep ravine,

under the skirts of a pine wood,
where the dead pine-leaves were our carpet,
and their tawny boughs stretched overhead.
But fire and smoke soon tamed the scene;
the rocks consented to be our walls,
and the pines our roof.[134]

Perhaps you visualized the scene. Did you really look down in the water and notice the clouds? Did you watch the muskrat swim by? Did you smell the wood fire? Did you feel tension in your arms during the paddling?

CHAPTER THIRTY-THREE

Mindfulness of Your Place in the Universe

I ONCE ATTENDED A SEVEN-DAY SILENT RETREAT at the Insight Meditation Society, a retreat center in central Massachusetts. Besides sitting meditation and walking meditation, there is not a lot to do, since besides not speaking, you're also asked not to read, text, or surf the internet during the retreat.

You can look at the sky. On some clear, moonless nights, I was able to find a dark place and lie back on the grass gazing up at the Milky Way.

The Milky Way is the hub of the galaxy that our sun inhabits. The sun is located on one of the spiral arms of the galaxy, so that when we look at the Milky Way, we are looking in from the suburbs, so to speak, to the central core of the galaxy. Even in fairly dark skies, the Milky Way is not that distinct. In fact, some years ago in a national park in Utah, I looked up at the night sky hoping to see the Milky Way. When I noticed a cloudy area just where it should be, I thought, "Just my luck. Clouds on the night I was hoping to see the Milky Way." But when the clouds didn't move, I realized they *were* the Milky Way!

Better informed now, I knew that the Milky Way could be found behind the Northern Cross in the constellation of Cygnus (the swan). And there it was, behind Cygnus, stretching all the way across the sky from the W-shaped constellation Cassiopeia to the "teapot" in Sagittarius.

As I gazed up at the Milky Way, I was mindful that I was a small creature looking out through space and past nearby stars to the center of our galaxy, and that my tiny body would be gravitationally pulled toward the center of this massive galaxy if it were not for the Earth's own gravity holding me firmly on the ground.

Exercise: Mindful Stargazing

You may not be able to see the Milky Way unless you are in a remote location without light pollution, but you should be able to see the major stars and some constellations if you can find a fairly dark spot away from streetlights. The clearest nights for stargazing are cold winter nights, but moonless summer nights are enjoyable too.

Be mindful of your personal safety. In some locations, it may be safest to do this exercise with a group. Bring a flashlight.

Before you go out, you may wish to prepare by studying a star guide or a book that shows you how to identify stars, such as H. A. Rey's *The Stars*. Rey, the creator of *Curious George*, provides a visual guide to help identify constellations and individual stars.

If it's a summer night, bring a blanket with you. Lay it down in a dark patch away from street lighting.

To get yourself into a meditative frame of mind, you may wish to do a few minutes of breath or sound meditation. It's best to do the meditation while sitting up so that you don't fall asleep. Once that's done, lie back on the blanket and look up at the sky.

As you gaze up at the sky, notice how your eyes gradually adjust to the dark, enabling you to see fainter stars.

Pick out a star group. If you are in the Northern Hemisphere, the Big Dipper will be visible on any clear night, unless it's obstructed by trees or buildings. The front two stars of the Big Dipper are a pointer that, if you follow it across the sky, leads you to the North Star. If you follow the pointer beyond the North Star, you come to the W-shaped constellation Cassiopeia. If you are looking at Cassiopeia, you are looking in the direction of the Milky Way, though whether you can see the Milky Way depends on lighting conditions in your area.

If you have binoculars, look at the sky through them. See how many faint stars are now visible that can't be seen with the naked eye.

While gazing at the stars, also notice the world around you. Notice the sound of leaves rustling in the wind. Notice the sound of crickets.

Notice your weight pressing you against the Earth.

Notice your place in the universe.

CHAPTER THIRTY-FOUR

Using Mindfulness to Break Bad Habits

PRACTICING MINDFULNESS can help you recognize habits and replace them with newer and better ones. This is a core element of mindfulness, and indeed why mindfulness is itself called a "practice."

As the story goes, after the Buddha's enlightenment, he was asked whether he was a god. He answered that he was not a god; rather, he was awake. In fact, the term *Buddha* means "Awakened One."[135]

What does it mean to be awake? Obviously, it doesn't mean that the Buddha was sleeping and just rolled out of bed. Rather, it means that he was not operating on what we would call "automatic pilot." In many respects, of course, the ability to do things automatically is a boon. Imagine having to pay attention to your feet *and* your jaw as you walk and chew gum. Somewhere back in our evolutionary history, the ability to multitask helped our ancestors survive. Without conscious thought we can perform skilled movements like walking and bicycling and more complex routines called habits.

Our conscious attention is a valuable and limited resource.

Our working memory — the part of our memory that deals with what is happening in the present moment — appears to have only one channel for sight and one for sound. Using any particular sense, we can pay attention to only one thing at a time. It's hard to listen to a conversation while you're listening to the radio, for instance.

Luckily, our ancestors evolved the ability to do many things without conscious attention. This is done by the brain's habit system. As rewards become predictable, the brain hands responsibility for the behaviors that produce them to the habit system, just as factory workers who do routine tasks can be replaced by machines.

Habits develop through repetition. The first time we do something — say, drive to a new job — we pay attention for fear of making a mistake or getting lost. But we don't pay as much attention driving to work the 249th time. The right turn after the Safeway becomes automatic.

If the habit system works unconsciously, and *you* don't deliberately choose to perform your habits, what does the choosing?

The psychologist Wendy Wood emphasizes that habits have triggers. "Most people think of their behavior as being internally driven," Wood told me. "We do things because we want to." But habits, she said, are triggered by something external — a familiar person, place, or thing. "It's the environment cuing the behavior," Wood said.

We may choose when to leave for work, but on a typical morning commute, we may be oblivious much of the time — at least until someone slams on the brakes ahead of us. "When something occurs that's unexpected, you come back to consciousness," she said.

Benjamin Franklin was perhaps the first American author to give advice on making and breaking habits. In his autobiography, Franklin identifies thirteen virtues that he wished to practice habitually, starting with moderation in eating and drinking. "I determined to give a week's strict attention to each of the virtues successively," Franklin writes.[136] Modern experts agree with Franklin on the importance of close attention when trying to change a habit.

Wendy Wood has studied people as they try to break habits. She says that becoming conscious of our automatic behavior is the key to overriding a habit. That's what mindfulness is: becoming aware of what we are doing, along with what is happening to us, in the present moment and with a spirit of kindness.

It's challenging, however, to pay attention to what we're doing all the time. Wood has found that people are more likely to relapse into old habits when they're tired or depleted. Similarly, in his 2011 book *Willpower*, the psychologist Roy Baumeister observes that conscious volition actually requires large amounts of glucose. The habit system, being automatic, requires less brain processing and less glucose. Thus, when our blood sugar is low, we're less able to exert willpower and more likely to fall back into automatic habits.[137]

Wood therefore sees conscious awareness not as something that can be maintained at all times, but as opening a brief window of opportunity to switch to a new and better habit. The MIT neuroscientist Ann Graybiel has found that traces of a habit take a long time to disappear. "Everyone always says that you cannot break a habit," Graybiel told me. "You've got to replace it with another habit."

Exercise: Breaking Bad Habits

Recognizing the habits you have is the first step in changing them. As you practice mindfulness in daily life, notice what you do. Notice when you do things you didn't consciously intend to do.

After you recognize a habit, investigate what may trigger that habit. Perhaps it's a time of day. For instance, most of us have bedtime rituals. By getting into a mindful state as you prepare for sleep, you may notice some habits you aren't fully aware of.

Sometimes being with other people triggers our habits. Perhaps there's something you've grown accustomed to doing when you are with one particular friend but with no one else. Sometimes it's a location that triggers a habit. If you walk home along a certain route, you'll stop at a bakery along the way and fall off your diet.

Once you are aware of a habit and aware of what triggers it, be mindful when the trigger is present and consciously choose a different behavior. For instance, you could cross the street before you reach the bakery and walk on the other side. If you repeat this new behavior with awareness a few times, it will start to become automatic.

The Robot inside Us

We often associate learning with memorizing facts and figures. There's another form of learning that psychologists call *implicit learning* because it happens unconsciously, managed by a collection of brain cells called the basal ganglia. Little by little, whatever we do leaves an imprint on the basal ganglia. The repetition of that imprinting is what turns behavior into a habit. Because this learning is unconscious, we can be unaware of our habits — until someone points them out to us.

When we consciously think through a task, we use what are called the executive functions of the brain. They act like a symphony conductor, telling the muscles that control our arms, legs, and other body parts when to come in. But just as an orchestra may eventually record its performance, the basal ganglia record our actions. Once we have a quality recording, we don't need a conductor.

Ann Graybiel has played a leading role in uncovering the role of the basal ganglia in developing habits. Researchers in Graybiel's lab at MIT study rats that have had electrodes implanted in their brains. When the rats are placed in a maze, they first sniff around, exploring their new surroundings. Eventually, they discover a reward, like a morsel of chocolate, at the end of the maze. The more times the experiment is repeated, the less the rats explore the maze, and the more they hustle to the end to find the chocolate. The process becomes almost automatic. Graybiel has found that once maze running becomes a habit, the cells in the rat's basal ganglia show a spike in activity at the start and end of the run. It looks as if the basal ganglia send "go" and "stop" signals to the parts of the brain that control the rat's muscles. Between the "go" and "stop," the muscles work robotically the way they've been trained.

When we do something routine, we think we're controlling it, but we're not, Graybiel says. She believes this applies not just to movements but also to habits of thought. To illustrate this point during my interview with her, she asked me what my office phone number was. I rattled off a string of digits.

"What's the fourth number?" she asked. I had to think for several seconds before I came up with "three."

She noticed my mental calculations and correctly pointed out that I had to run through the sequence of numbers to get to the one I wanted. "You've got it so packaged that you can't get inside."

A habit, in other words, is a sequence of thoughts and movements that have been recorded, packaged, and shrink-wrapped. It's sometimes better to accept this package and trust your habit rather than trying to control it consciously. "That's what anybody who has tried to learn a backhand has learned with humbling experience," Graybiel said. "You simply cannot think about each little part, because if you do you screw it up."

CHAPTER THIRTY-FIVE

Making a Habit of Mindfulness

MAKING MINDFULNESS A HABIT seems paradoxical: habits are things that we do automatically and with little attention, whereas mindfulness is about paying attention to the present moment. Yet we can develop a habit of paying attention to the present.

One purpose of meditation practice is to cultivate habits. Josh Bartok, a Zen priest who leads a *sangha*, or Buddhist community, in Boston, says that meditation practice is just that. "It isn't a matter of blissing out or being relaxed," he told me. "It is *literally* practice, as you might go to a batting cage to practice your swing. You practice in the easy situations of special time, special place, special cushions." Then you can apply your meditative practice when it really counts — in day-to-day living. Practice makes you more mindful and compassionate in less accommodating situations.

It's been said, "You do not rise to the occasion. You sink to the level of your training."[138] If you want to cultivate mindfulness, you've got to practice. Keep practicing until it becomes the habit that you fall back on when you are under stress.

The Buddhist teacher Narayan Helen Liebenson told me that even in stressful moments that push our emotional buttons, reacting with kindness can become a habit if we cultivate it. "In that moment — this is where practice comes in — we're able to remember. *Metta* becomes our fallback instead of ill-will being our fallback or instead of confusion being our fallback," she said.

Practice also makes behaviors easier to do by strengthening brain areas involved in the task. Sara Lazar's research team at Massachusetts General Hospital found that an eight-week mindfulness-based stress reduction course resulted in measurable changes in the gray matter of the brain — the brain cells that do much of the work in processing thoughts and feelings. Practice can lead to physical changes in the wiring of the brain, a phenomenon also known as *neuroplasticity*.[139]

Despite the paradox of developing an automatic habit of paying attention, I have developed certain mindfulness habits. For instance, I have practiced mindful dishwashing enough times that when I'm standing in front of the kitchen sink, I think without prompting, "Oh, opportunity for mindfulness." And then I wash the dishes mindfully, without having planned to do so. If I drive to a nearby hiking trail, I might be a little distracted during the drive, but once I have my boots on, I think, "Hey, I can be mindful," and it comes. So being in certain locations now triggers my mindfulness habit and wakes me up from whatever reverie I've been in.

Exercise: Making Mindfulness a Habit

To develop a habit of mindfulness, it's more important to practice frequently than to practice for a long time. The habit will become more ingrained if you meditate every day for five minutes than once a week for forty-five minutes.

In cultivating good habits, we can take advantage of the fact that the habit system works by means of triggers.[140] Because habits are triggered by locations, it can help to have a special place for meditation. It should be a place that you pass by frequently enough that it reminds you to meditate regularly.

Because habits are also triggered by time of day, it can help to set a special time to meditate. A few minutes in the morning or around lunchtime can become a habit. Many people use the trigger of a phone ringing to take a mindful breath.

If you only have time for brief meditations on most days, a longer meditation once a week can help you deepen your practice. Being part of a group that meets regularly is a good way to incorporate it into your schedule. If your meditation practice doesn't settle into a slot somewhere in your routine, it's likely to fizzle out.

But even if you can't find time to meditate, it is certainly possible to integrate mindfulness and loving-kindness practices into your daily routine. You can practice loving-kindness toward coworkers and people you see on the street (whether you tell them about it is another story). You can walk mindfully, noticing the space around you, the sounds and the light.

You can select events to serve as triggers for informal practice. For instance, if practicing loving-kindness toward everyone seems burdensome, you can practice it the first time each day that you walk by someone you don't know. If your mornings are too busy for mindful dishwashing, you can mindlessly stuff the breakfast dishes into the dishwasher. But after a relaxed dinner, try washing the dishes mindfully — or just the forks.

Habits Provide Little Reward

The advantage of habits is that they require little or no attention; the disadvantage is they provide little or no reward. Because we're not aware of what we're doing, we miss out on the pleasure of doing it. This is what happens when we take things for granted.

We become more aware when things are different from what we expect. The reward system responds most keenly to *novelty*. The Emory University psychiatrist Gregory Berns scanned the brains of test subjects who were offered squirts of fruit juice. He found that the reward system responds most actively when squirts come at intervals that are hard to predict. The neuroscientist Wolfram Schultz of Cambridge University and Paul Glimcher, director of the Center for Neuroeconomics at New York University, have studied this phenomenon at the level of individual brain cells. They find that dopamine-sensitive neurons respond best when rewards are unexpected.[141]

By paying closer attention, we notice new and unexpected things. This novelty activates the reward system. By restoring a sense of freshness to everyday routines, mindfulness can make daily life more rewarding.

CHAPTER THIRTY-SIX

Other Frequently Asked Questions

What's with this label "secular Buddhism"? It sounds like another religion.

That label is shorthand that helps people quickly understand that we've taken things from Buddhism but secularized them. And although our meditations are mostly derived from Buddhism, mantra meditation is really a secularization of Hindu practice.

Over 2,500 years, Asian civilizations have come up with some good ideas. Even as India and the Far East are increasingly becoming Westernized, it's fitting for Westerners to Easternize by assimilating the best of Asian learning.

Aside from the supernatural elements, there are other aspects of Buddhist philosophy — such as notions about the self — that may or may not be true. Moreover, just like other claims within the realm of science — for instance, the claim that a low-fat diet prevents heart disease — claims that Buddhist ideas comport with neuroscience have to be carefully assessed. The bottom line is that we find a great deal of value in Buddhism, but we don't have faith in Buddhism, nor do we even give it the benefit of the doubt. We are experimenting with it, evaluating it, and assimilating those practices and ideas that seem beneficial and valid according to secular standards.

Some Buddhists have criticized secular Buddhism because they think it waters down Buddhism. I like to think of it as adding Buddhist flavoring to the sparkling water of secularism. Personally, I do not consider myself to be Buddhist but rather "Buddhist-ish." Others in the secular Buddhist community may fully embrace a Buddhist identity. But one valuable piece of Buddhist wisdom is not to cling to identities but to hold on to them lightly. In that spirit, our embrace of Buddhism is light and affectionate, not a tight grip.

Do you put the Buddha on some sort of pedestal?

We see the Buddha as being more of a philosopher like Socrates than a religious prophet like Jesus. In this, we follow the point of view of Stephen Batchelor, a former Buddhist monk who is a leading voice in secular Buddhism. Batchelor is the author of the books *Buddhism Without Beliefs* and *Confession of a Buddhist Atheist*. He has spoken to the Humanist Community at Harvard twice, and I once enjoyed the privilege of having dinner with him.

According to Batchelor, the Buddha was certainly agnostic about the gods worshipped in India and quite possibly was an atheist.[142] Like others of his time, however, he did believe in rebirth. We humanists think he was mistaken on this point. In Greece, Plato appears to have believed in a somewhat analogous doctrine of the transmigration of souls, and yet we have no trouble thinking of Plato as a philosopher rather than a religious figure. Batchelor suggests that there's evidence that the Buddha had some secondhand exposure to Greek ideas, which had reached India during his lifetime.

Is humanism a religion?

Humanism is a philosophy of life but not a religion. Both religion and philosophy are ways for people to find direction and meaning in the world. So, in that sense, humanism is like a religion, but without any supernatural belief.

Because it relies on human understanding, which is fallible, humanism makes no claims to absolute truth. Humanism seeks to embrace all human beings within its circle of concern, rather than just those who self-identify as humanists. And just because the label refers to our own species, it doesn't mean we don't care about other species.

Why should I trust what you've written?

I encourage you to be skeptical of everything I've written here. Many humanists are involved with the skeptical movement, which is made up of people who try to debunk pseudoscience and other claims that have little or no evidence to support them. This is a worthwhile effort. But I would encourage skeptics to distinguish between theory and practice. Eastern religions contain some questionable ideas, such as rebirth, but this is not necessarily a reason to dismiss everything connected with Eastern religion. Sometimes practices work even if the theory that goes along with them is incorrect.

For example, the bacteria *Yersinia pestis* is responsible for bubonic plague. It is believed to have spread from Central Asia and been responsible for the Black Death that devastated Europe in the 1300s. The bacteria had long persisted in the marmot population of Manchuria. Yet the native peoples were little affected, perhaps because trapping of these rodents was taboo due to certain cultural myths. In the early twentieth century, Chinese immigrants into Manchuria scorned the native superstitions and began to trap the marmot for its fur. The result was an outbreak of plague that spread from the countryside to cities along railway lines. The theory behind avoiding marmots had no basis in science, but the practice was sound.[143]

At the Humanist Mindfulness Group, we take an empirical approach. We try out practices to see if they work, even if we don't quite know *why* they work. Based on our personal experiences, it seems that many of these practices are helpful. We've gained further confidence that this pursuit is worthwhile as more and more scientific studies demonstrate benefits from meditation and mindfulness. These studies are being done in respected academic settings and published in legitimate, peer-reviewed journals.

As to how meditation works, it's still a bit of a puzzle. Increasingly, though, the pieces are coming together. Researchers at Emory University have scanned the brains of people doing a twenty-minute breath meditation and identified the brain systems active when the meditators concentrated on the breath, became distracted, noticed their distraction, and returned to the breath. The brain areas active when subjects were distracted included areas associated with spontaneous inner speech and self-referential thoughts.[144] Focusing on the breath deactivates these brain areas, a finding that could account for the subjective experience that meditation quiets inner chatter and reduces self-oriented ruminations.

In addition to the changes that occur while meditating, there is evidence that meditation leads to long-term changes in the brain. Researchers led by Sara Lazar at Massachusetts General Hospital, which is associated with Harvard Medical School, have shown that an eight-week mindfulness meditation class leads to structural changes in brain areas related to emotional regulation and self-referential thinking. Richie Davidson and colleagues at the University of Wisconsin have used brain scans to investigate how compassion meditation affects empathetic responses to suffering. They found signs of greater responsiveness in the brains of long-term meditators.[145]

There is a lot of evidence that meditation and mindfulness can be helpful. But like anything humans do, it can be overhyped and oversold, so we encourage people to retain their skepticism.

Why meditate? Why not just go into therapy if you are having emotional problems?

This isn't an either/or choice. You can do both if it's appropriate. Recently, meditation and mindfulness have generated a lot of interest within the psychotherapy community. There is an Institute for Meditation and Psychotherapy in the Boston area; its former president, the psychotherapist Paul Fulton, gave a talk to our group. Even if you have an established meditation practice, you may encounter personal losses that can't simply be meditated away. You should not be reluctant to seek the help of a therapist in such cases.

In many cases, however, a person's suffering doesn't rise to the level that requires treatment by a medical professional. Freud wrote that the goal of his treatment was to turn a patient's deep misery into "common unhappiness."[146] Meditation and mindfulness can help us deal with this common unhappiness through practices that can shift our emotions in a fairly direct manner.

Why bother with cultivating emotions? Why not just be logical?

Logic helps us maximize what we value, but it cannot tell us *what* we value. The neurologist Antonio Damasio, at the University of Southern California, has argued that people can't reason effectively without emotion: we simply don't have the brainpower. Emotions help us set limits to our rational calculations. In his 1994 book *Descartes' Error*, Damasio discusses patients with damage to parts of the brain necessary to feel emotions. Free of emotion but with their logical faculties intact, one might expect them to make cool, efficient decisions. Instead, his ultrarational patients suffered from a sort of "analysis paralysis." They dithered, exploring rational choices beyond the point of diminishing returns.[147] To know what you want, you have to have feelings.

Logic tells us that two apples are better than one — if we accept that more is better. Logic cannot tell us whether an apple is better than a tomato, and it's entirely debatable whether two Brussels sprouts are better than one.

Even being rational has a *feel* to it. Those who enjoy math feel delight when they prove a theorem, and distress on discovering an error in their work.

The humanist creator of *Star Trek*, Gene Roddenberry, understood that logic is of significant yet finite use. Mr. Spock was not the show's main character. To be at our best, we must use not only our logical and analytical intelligences but also our emotional intelligence. Freedom and equality are not values that can be deduced from the laws of physics. Even the biological sciences are of questionable value as a guide to morality, having been used in the past to justify hierarchy and discrimination. Our deepest values stem, in fact, from feelings, such as the desire to understand nature and empathy for living beings that suffer.

We can sometimes guess why we like apples, cute animals, or lovers, but we can't explain it logically; feelings of desire and satisfaction arise in areas of the brain such as the reward system that are not accessible to conscious introspection. We can attempt to justify subjective choices by logical means: the young Charles Darwin, for instance, made a written list of the pros and cons of marriage. Among the pros he listed "Charms of music and female chit-chat," and among the advantages of not marrying, "Conversation of clever men at clubs."[148] But analyses like Darwin's can only advance so far before they rest on evaluations — like how much one values conversation and music — that are based entirely on feelings.

Just as our desires are nonlogical, so are our aversions. Prominent in aversion is a brain area called the insula, which is involved with visceral feelings in the body, especially from the gastrointestinal system. Desire motivates us to approach objects; disgust pushes us away from them. These gut feelings can, in fact, provide worthwhile information. In the book *Blink*, Malcolm Gladwell describes international art experts who felt an "intuitive repulsion" when viewing an ancient Greek statue. This unexpected emotion led them to question its authenticity, and a subsequent audit of acquisition records showed it to be a modern forgery.[149]

If we discarded emotion, we'd eliminate desire, aversion, and preference. Without the brain's reward system, we would not be motivated to eat, move, or speak. People with Asperger syndrome have brain deficits that force them to intellectually puzzle out social behavior that comes naturally to most of us as we perceive the emotions of others. That's not something to be envied.

For many or perhaps most people, many basic decisions are emotional; we come up with logical reasons after the fact.[150] To make truly rational decisions, it helps to be mindful of our actual emotional state. For instance, if we hate someone, we're unlikely to think rationally about them. Having the skill to shift our emotions at least to a more neutral attitude can help us think more clearly.

Love is not *all* we need, but neither is reason. It is the combination of the two that holds the best prospects for relieving suffering and improving well-being, which is the proper aim of a humanistic community.

Doesn't secularization take away the poetry?

It's true that our initial attempts at articulating a secular philosophy may result in using language that is less poetic than the texts and rituals of spiritual traditions that are centuries old. In the shift toward gender-neutral language some years ago, the initial approach was to replace the word *man* with *person*, leading to such monstrosities as *fireperson*.[151] Eventually a more poetic term, *firefighter*, was popularized that is both gender neutral and satisfying. So the poetry may come in time.

In the meantime, we believe that adopting secular language is important for the sake of clarity. For instance, people often casually use the word *karma* as shorthand for the belief that when you do something improper, it can come back to bite you. But *karma* can also be taken to refer to a sort of supernatural accounting system that punishes people for their sins over multiple lifetimes. We prefer not to use language that might carry this kind of connotation, even if it sounds cool.

Should I meditate alone or in a group?

You can certainly meditate on your own, but a group can offer valuable support. If you always meditate alone, you may be more inclined to slack off. Being part of a group can encourage you to continue your practice. It can also boost your confidence in meditation in the face of skepticism from others that might make you wonder if it's a little weird.

Meditation and mindfulness are practical skills, and even though you can learn certain things from books, it can be helpful to see how other people do it. To make progress, it helps to share experiences with others. If you are having difficulties with your meditation, hearing about other people's challenges can reassure you that it's not that you're incompetent and should give up, but rather that it takes a while to develop these skills. It's also useful to see that some people have a harder time with some meditations than others. Knowing this can help you find meditations that suit your personal style.

Where can I find a meditation group?

If you like the secular approach I've presented here, you might look for a group with similar beliefs and values. Unfortunately, there are not many of these, but you can find a listing through the Secular Buddhist Association. I have also joined online meditations sponsored by the Secular Buddhist Association that included participants across North America and even Australia. In the resources section, I list websites that can be helpful. You are, of course, invited to drop by the Humanist Community at Harvard if you are in the Boston area.

Many congregations affiliated with the Unitarian Universalist Association host meditation groups; these are often but not always secular. If there are no secular meditations in your area, you might consider starting a group of your own. We have found that our listing on Meetup.com is an effective way to attract new members.

If that seems too ambitious, you might try going to a Buddhist center that is not strictly secular but fairly low-key in its approach. I have benefited from attending workshops associated with the Insight Meditation approach. Many secular Buddhists have benefited from training in Zen Buddhism.

Are there any physical health benefits to meditation?

A number of studies of varying quality have been published showing health benefits from meditation. In 2014, *JAMA Internal Medicine* published a systematic review of forty-seven studies with 3,515 participants. It found evidence that mindfulness meditation programs had a small positive impact in helping people deal with anxiety, depression, and physical pain. There was no evidence that they did any harm. Neither was there evidence that meditation worked better than alternatives such as behavioral therapy or pharmaceutical drugs.[152] So really, it's up to individuals to determine what works best for them.

Are there any risks associated with meditation?

Just because meditation is "natural" and does not involve the ingestion of drugs doesn't mean it can't have negative effects. It's unlikely that a twenty-minute meditation like the ones presented here will cause such problems. But meditators on long retreats that involve days of silence and isolation have occasionally developed mental illnesses that require professional treatment.[153] So if you have any history of mental health problems or trauma, exercise caution and seek out a good teacher as you start to meditate.

One reason negative effects may occur is that, while meditation seems to deactivate brain areas responsible for stress, it may also deactivate brain areas that repress traumatic memories. The psychiatrist Michael Grodin, cofounder of the Boston Center for Refugee Health and Human Rights, has treated refugee Tibetan monks who were tortured in China. Grodin said in an interview with *Bostonia* magazine that the monks suffered from posttraumatic stress disorder and sometimes had flashbacks during meditation. He said, "I think the Tibetans doing higher-level meditation were having a disinhibition: their frontal lobes were keeping a hold on things, but when they got into this deep meditative state, all kinds of bad experiences and feelings came out."[154]

The Brown University neuroscientist Willoughby Britton, who is a meditation practitioner, warns that most advanced practitioners face challenging side effects along the way. These can include anxiety, mood changes, and awareness of unusual bodily sensations. "It does seem to be the case that the longer that you practice and the more intensely that you practice that these types of experiences seemed to be the norm," she told Vincent Horn in an interview for the *Buddhist Geeks* podcast.[155]

When I asked the psychiatrist Daniel Siegel about possible negative side effects of meditation, he said:

> I've asked the exact same question, concerned that at least we "do no harm." The answers I've gotten are this: in short-term ways of focusing on the breath or focusing on

something internally for a few minutes, there is no negative side effect and there is no condition for which that's a problem. Even for someone with psychosis, three, four minutes of inward focusing where you're present with them — they can come right out of it and talk to you about it. That's what I've been told by professionals in the field. For long, extended meditations, that can become problematic, and for week-long silent retreats, it can become extremely problematic because the brain is a very social organ and it requires social communication to maintain its sense of equilibrium.... For these longer ones, we want to really be careful.

Herbert Benson warns against meditating for too long in *The Relaxation Response*. Benson writes, "From our personal observations, many people who meditate for several hours every day for weeks at a time tend to hallucinate." Benson wrote that he'd never observed such a side effect in people who practiced meditation for ten to twenty minutes at a time once or twice a day.[156]

Treat meditation as a form of exercise. Trying to bench-press too much weight can lead to injury. Sitting quietly for twenty minutes is unlikely to harm you. But if you have little experience, meditating for long periods can be risky. It's wise to build up a meditation practice slowly, and ideally in a community with other people.

If you meditate and you experience disturbing thoughts, stop. Instead of meditating on your own, seek the guidance of an experienced teacher.

Can meditation help you live longer?

There is an old joke about an Englishman who went to see a Tibetan lama who knew the secret of eternal life. The Englishman sailed to India and climbed high into the Himalayas to reach Tibet. Finally, he found the cave where the lama lived in seclusion. He apologized to the lama for interrupting his meditation and asked him if he knew the secret to eternal life.

"Yes," said the lama.

"What must I do?" asked the Englishman.

"First, you must not smoke," said the lama.

"I'll quit my pipe right away," promised the Englishman.

"Next, you must not drink alcohol or any intoxicants," said the lama.

"I'll try to do that," said the Englishman.

"Finally, you must abstain from all sexual relations," said the lama.

"Hmmm," the Englishman wondered. "If I do, will I live forever?"

"Maybe not," said the lama. "But it will sure seem that way."

Science-based meditation started with medically based programs such as Benson's Relaxation Response and the Mindfulness-Based Stress Reduction Program at the University of Massachusetts Medical School. There is a lot of evidence that these programs help people reduce stress.[157] Conceivably, then, meditation may prolong life by protecting against stress-linked illnesses such as heart disease.

Even more intriguingly, a recent study found that participants in an intensive three-month meditation retreat showed greater activity of an enzyme that protects against cell aging. There is also some evidence from Sara Lazar's lab that meditation may protect against the thinning of the cerebral cortex that comes with aging and thus protect against cognitive decline.[158]

On the other hand, just as the practice of loving-kindness does not preclude you from locking the front door of your home, the practice of mindfulness should not make you complacent about risks to your health. A study of older adults in Germany found that pessimists lived longer than optimists and had less disability. One interpretation of the results is that pessimists take more precautions about their health and safety.[59] As we've discussed, the nonjudgmental aspect of mindfulness is about muting *emotional* judgments, not about eliminating rational decision making. The message of mindfulness — accepting what is going on at present with a friendly attitude — should not be taken to the point where someone becomes overly accepting of symptoms that could indicate a serious health problem.

If you are mindful and pay attention to what is going on in the present moment, you will be more aware of what you eat and how it may affect your health. You'll be more aware of your exposure to risk in a variety of situations. Mindfulness has the potential to help people live healthy and long lives, but whether it actually does is not yet known.

Is there anything else in Buddhism that you'd like to assimilate into secular culture?

In Buddhist tradition, the Four Noble Truths are part of the first discourse that the Buddha delivered shortly after his "enlightenment" to five disciples at the Deer Park near Varanasi, India. These Four Noble Truths purport to describe the origin of and solution to suffering. As secularists, we don't believe in Truth with a capital *T*. Everything we know comes from human observation, and human beings can be wrong. But the Four Noble Truths — or at least the first three of them — can be seen as valid and valuable from a secular perspective.

Unlike the Bible's Ten Commandments, the Four Noble Truths are not attributed to a supernatural source. The Buddha arrived at them through self-examination. They can be expressed as follows:

1. Life comes with suffering, including physical pain and mental anguish.
2. Suffering comes from desiring things to be other than as they are — wanting what we don't have or having what we don't want.
3. Relief comes from detachment from this desire.
4. The way to achieve this relief is to follow a set of ethical principles and mental attitudes known as the Eightfold Path.

What's nice about the Four Noble Truths is that they are testable hypotheses. The first three Noble Truths are consistent with the findings of contemporary neuroscience; the fourth is plausible, though not fully tested.

Few will argue with the first noble truth — that life is full of suffering. It's not that life is nothing but suffering, but rather that suffering goes with the territory. The second is a little less obvious, but it's consistent with what neuroscientists have learned about the brain's salience network — the network of brain regions that monitor how we're doing compared to our goals. The feeling of suffering is in essence a signal that we're off track. When a gap opens up between our goals and reality, we get a negative feedback signal. That's what suffering is — a signal that motivates us to act to change our present reality.

The second noble truth, however, warns us that clinging to unattainable goals increases our suffering. Reya Stevens is a practitioner of Theravada Buddhism who teaches Buddhist approaches to illness. "Clinging," she told me, "is all about not wanting something to be the way it is, or wanting something to stay the way it is — which can't happen, because everything is constantly changing." It's natural to reject what's unpleasant, but this often has a boomerang effect. "If you get into a struggle with something, like try to get rid of something or push it away, it has a tendency to actually make the thing worse," she said.

If trying to suppress something negative has the ironic effect of magnifying it, can accepting it actually alleviate suffering? This insight is the basis of the third noble truth. If instead of rejecting a negative event, you observe it without emotional judgment, your sense of alarm diminishes. By accepting the present reality — which is what mindfulness entails — you are instructing the salience network that what is happening right now is *not* in conflict with your immediate goals. If there is no conflict, no need for negative feedback to spur us to action, the salience network no longer generates the feeling of suffering.

The fourth noble truth is that the solution to suffering comes from following what Buddhists call the Eightfold Path. This has eight elements:

right view
right intention
right speech
right action
right livelihood
right effort
right mindfulness
right concentration

In broad terms, the fourth noble truth says that one should think with intelligence and care, act accordingly, and cultivate mental practices like meditation and mindfulness. At this level, I think the Eightfold Path is compatible with humanism and provides a reasonably secular vision of ethics, along with a valid approach to easing suffering.

In the details, however, some aspects of Buddhist philosophy and humanist philosophy might be at odds. For instance, the traditional Buddhist view of right speech discourages speech that may be hurtful even if true. Yet investigative journalism is based on ferreting out information that is negative but true, which might be hurtful to an individual but beneficial to society as a whole. Thus, although ethical behavior is important in order to relieve suffering, the specifics of the Buddhist ethical code may need some updating for the twenty-first century.

Are traditional Buddhist views of enlightenment credible?

I'm skeptical that enlightenment is all it's cracked up to be. In the book *Zen at War*, Brian Victoria discusses how Zen masters supported Japanese militarism before and during World War II; these individuals were considered enlightened by their contemporaries. The Dalai Lama has condemned attacks on Muslim minorities in majority-Buddhist countries that were reportedly incited by Buddhist monks. Over the past few years, a number of scandals involving Buddhist teachers, often of a sexual nature, have come to light.[160] There's no reason to think the problem is any worse in Buddhism than in any other religion, but neither is there much reason to think it's any better. These incidents raise the question of whether the pursuit of enlightenment has an ethical component or is just a sort of mental athleticism.

The pursuit of enlightenment has always been an elite practice in Buddhist societies. In the past, a small number of meditative monks were supported by laypeople who provided them with food and other support. The reward for these "householders" was merit that would benefit them in a future life. Aside from the supernaturalism embedded in this model, it doesn't seem that Buddhist intentions to reduce suffering were all that effectively translated into concrete actions that reduced suffering in society at large. Many contemporary Buddhist societies are quite poor in economic terms. Arguably, science and technology have done more to relieve the suffering of poor people than meditation has.

Still, I think there's evidence that "enlightenment" is a special brain state. In the book *Zen and the Brain*, James Austin, a professor of neurology and a longtime Zen practitioner, describes his own experience of *kensho*, a dropping away of the sense of self. Eight years after starting to practice Zen, Austin experienced it for less than a minute before it retreated from his consciousness. As he describes it, he experienced a profound loss of the sense of being an *I*, a self separate from the rest of the world. It typically takes many years of training for Buddhist monks to experience this awareness.[161]

Sam Harris, the author of *Waking Up*, came to the Humanist Community at Harvard to discuss his conclusion that the feeling of having a self, an *I*, is an illusion. Based on personal experience, he says that cutting through this illusion is deeply rewarding. Harris's years of experience with meditation, as well as his dedication to secularism, give him a great deal of credibility. He makes a strong case that the sense of self is just another thing the brain does, rather than an essential component of consciousness.[162]

Harris and Austin clearly think that achieving this sense of egolessness is a good thing. Their experiences, however, must be classified (but not dismissed) as anecdotal. We are nowhere near having statistical evidence that tells us whether the state of nonself leads to a better quality of life or to compassion for others.[163]

The neuroscientist and meditation practitioner Willoughby Britton said in a *Buddhist Geeks* podcast that many practitioners experience the dropping away of their sense of self as disturbing:

> Even though you can read about this and think that this might be the goal of the contemplative path, for a lot of people it's very, very scary when that happens. And so

what I mean by a drop in the sense of self, it can be a lack of a feeling like there's anybody controlling. So when words are coming out of the mouth, like who would be speaking them? When you move your arms and legs and walk, it's not really sure who decided that. When somebody asks you a question, there's almost a panicked feeling because you don't know who's going to answer the question. There's a sort of temporal disintegration. So your sense of time can fall apart, along with your sense of a narrative self over time. Part of the sense of self is about being able to have continuity over time. And if you just don't have that kind of sense of past and future and you only have a sense of now, your sense of self just by not having a past and a future and being able to imagine that can be sort of truncated and attenuated.[164]

I see selflessness or non-self as more of a direction to head toward rather than a destination we can expect to reach. Loving-kindness practice is a concrete means to move in this direction, to help raise empathy and lower the barriers of concern between people and between nations. I prefer to cultivate a shift of perspective from *I* to *we* rather than from *I* to *non-self*. This can also help us get out of the trap of evaluating our lives based on personal goals that might not be achievable. Instead, we can identify with a larger purpose and experience sympathetic joy as we progress together toward our goals.

For now, at least, our focus in the Humanist Mindfulness Group is to cultivate evidence-based practices that the average person can pursue with a reasonable likelihood of success in a modest amount of time. We don't discourage members of our group from pursuing the more advanced Buddhist practices that lead to the brain state called enlightenment, but we do encourage them to maintain a skeptical outlook as they experiment.

What do you think of as enlightenment?

I like an approach discussed by Thanissaro Bhikkhu, an American Theravada Buddhist monk. He writes about training the mind to get to a point at which one's happiness is not dependent on conditions in the world but instead comes from within.[165]

The goal, as I see it, would be to cultivate an ability to love that is not just a momentary state but a character trait. Happiness would not depend on achieving success in the world. If that were to come, it would be gravy, but internally generated love is the main dish. Similarly, inevitable losses, including those due to aging and death, could be absorbed with equanimity, because our internally generated sense of love is larger than those losses.

Trying to force equanimity leads to apathy and disguised depression. But if you can train yourself in mindfulness and loving-kindness, so that they become highly rewarding, then extrinsic rewards like money and fame become minor compared to the satisfaction you already feel. Likewise, you don't need to cling to the trappings of success and prestige, for even if you lose them, you will be fine inside yourself. I have not achieved this level of equanimity myself, but it's the direction I aim toward. I am not happy at every moment, but I'm happiest when I remember to focus on the present moment with a spirit of loving-kindness.

Tips on Creating Your Own Mindfulness Group

1. Hook up with existing national groups, such as those listed in the resources section below. They may know of other people in your area interested in forming a group.
2. Use a social networking site to organize. Although the Humanist Mindfulness Group gets some attention through Facebook, we have found that most newcomers learn of us through Meetup.com, which lists groups and activities by locality.
3. Find free or low-cost space. In the summer, you may be able to meditate in a park or other outdoor area. At other times, you may find that a school or community organization will allow you to meet in their space.
4. Try to find a regular time to meet, so that people can work it into their schedules and make it a habit.
5. Be welcoming, but also be clear. In our group we welcome newcomers and briefly explain to them our humanistic philosophy. Sometimes people with supernaturalistic beliefs come to check us out. We are friendly and don't try to argue with them about their

beliefs, but we do state the guiding principles of our group in clear and positive terms.

6. Give instructions, but don't talk too much either. Providing instructions before starting a meditation is useful as an introduction for new people and a reminder for others. But don't talk too much: people are there for a meditation, not a lecture.

7. Practice compassionate and mindful speech. Many secular groups are plagued by friction and angry splits. Although arguments can be stimulating, discussions should be conducted in a way that incorporates loving-kindness and keeps people feeling connected to each other.

8. Encourage people to speak about their emotions and respect their confidences. Don't offer advice unless it's been requested. Make sure everyone has a chance to speak, but don't require people to speak. Secular groups often feature lectures and highly intellectual discussions. These can be enjoyable, but life is more than that. A mindfulness group is a place where people can open up about their emotional lives and find support.

9. Socialize afterward. People will show up for the meditations, but they'll keep coming back when they find they can relate to the people in the group. Going out to eat afterward has helped many members of our group get to know and like each other.

A Secular Invocation

POLITICAL SPEECH IN THE UNITED STATES seems to be increasingly toxic — quite the opposite of compassionate speech. One opportunity for setting a compassionate tone is to offer an invocation before public meetings. I offer the following as an example of a secular invocation:

> We are in this space to further the public good. We have different perspectives because each of us has had different life experiences. To help us love — or at least not despise — our opponents, let's take a moment to summon feelings of love and kindness.
>
> Let us all think of a person who really helped us at some point in our life. When we think of this person, we feel warmth and gratitude. If we can, let's visualize this person in our imagination and look upon them with eyes filled with kindness and love.
>
> Even with loved ones, we sometimes disagree, but we find a way to work out our differences. Let us bring this same spirit to our dealings with the people we encounter here.

Let us also remember that not everyone in our community is present here. Let us be considerate of the interests of those who are absent and also of the interests of those not yet born who may live in this community someday.

Finally, let us breathe in and breathe out, and when anger rises, remember to take a breath before speaking, so that we are reasonable people engaged in dialogue.

Acknowledgments

THIS BOOK WOULD NOT HAVE BEEN POSSIBLE without the participation and support of the Humanist Community at Harvard and especially its director, Greg Epstein, who has provided critical support at every step. Thanks to the staff as well, including Sarah Chandonnet, Jade Meshasha, and Christopher Raiche.

Thanks to the members of the Humanist Mindfulness Group, and especially to those who provided feedback for this book, including David, Doug, Jennifer, Kieran, Laura, Laurie, Marc, and Steven. Thanks to Forrest for encouraging us to daydream. Thanks to Molly for introducing us to *metta* meditation and to Paul for his help in the early years. Thanks especially to Pat for her extraordinary work in closely reviewing the manuscript.

Thanks to Zach Alexander, who founded the Humanist Mindfulness Group, following a trail blazed by D. T. Strain in Houston. Strain and B. T. Newberg of the Spiritual Naturalist Society provided helpful feedback for this book. Thanks to Sam Harris for making meditation respectable among humanists and to Stephen Batchelor for making secularism respectable among Buddhists.

Thanks to Tim Kiely, who founded the Cambridge Secular Buddhists, which later merged with the Humanist Mindfulness

Group. He was inspired by Ted Meissner and the Secular Buddhist Association. At the SBA, Ted, Mark Knickelbine, and others have created a space where Buddhist ideas can be explored in a secular context.

I have learned a great deal from attending meditations and workshops at the Cambridge Insight Meditation Center, and in particular from the teachers Narayan Helen Liebenson, Michael Grady, and Maddy Klyne. Thanks also to visiting teachers, including Jack Kornfield and Chas DiCapua.

Thanks to the staff and teachers at the Barre Center for Buddhist Studies and the Insight Meditation Society.

Thanks to the Arlington Center and the Institute for Meditation and Psychotherapy. Thanks to Christopher Germer and Kristin Neff for their workshop on self-compassion.

Thanks to the scientists and researchers who have advanced my understanding of the brain in connection with meditation, mindfulness, and compassion, including Kent Berridge, Barbara Fredrickson, Tim Gard, Ann Graybiel, Stephen Grossberg, Catherine Kerr, Ellen Langer, Sara Lazar, Paul Lehrer, Dan Siegel, Michael Spezio, Wendy Wood, and Paul Zak.

Thanks to Rick Hanson, whose workshops were important in advancing my understanding of the intersection of neuroscience and meditative practice. Rick was pivotal in bringing me together with New World Library.

Thanks to Jennifer Bardi, Josh Bartok, David Chernikoff, Tynette Deveaux, Scott Earnshaw, James Ishmael Ford, Poh Lim, Doug Muder, Chris Walton, and Shinzen Young.

Thanks to Jason Gardner and Erika Büky at New World Library.

Zachary Bos provided extremely useful ideas to help me structure this book.

Thanks to Jonathan Bellot for making me familiar with defamiliarization.

Thanks to Boston's Grub Street. Thanks to Katie Willis-Morton for suggestions on both form and content.

Thanks to Herbert Benson for pioneering a secular approach to meditation; to Jon Kabat-Zinn for creating the Mindfulness-Based Stress Reduction program, which has provided much of the evidentiary basis that has opened the minds of secular people with regard to meditation; to Sharon Salzberg for her emphasis on loving-kindness meditation; and to Thanissaro Bhikkhu for his translations.

Thanks to Cindy, my wife and companion, who has supported my writing for many, many years.

Resources

Personal

My website is www.rickheller.com.
You can follow me on Twitter at @secularmeditate.

Humanist Community at Harvard, www.humanisthub.org

The Humanist Community at Harvard meets at the "Humanist Hub" in Harvard Square, Cambridge, Massachusetts, and is open to everyone. We hold regular meditations, and you are invited to join us if you are in the area.

Other Secular-Friendly Resources

Buddhist Geeks, www.buddhistgeeks.com

Buddhist Geeks is an innovative community for Buddhists with an interest in digital technology. Many, though not all, have secular leanings. The community is mostly online but has hosted real-world conferences.

Center for Mindfulness, www.umassmed.edu/cfm/

This is the home of the Mindfulness-Based Stress Reduction program. The program is entirely secular. Participants come from a wide variety of backgrounds.

Institute for Meditation and Psychotherapy, meditationandpsychotherapy.org

The institute provides training chiefly for mental health professionals seeking to integrate mindfulness practice with psychotherapy.

Secular Buddhist Association, secularbuddhism.org

The Secular Buddhist Association is an online community for people who approach Buddhist practice from a naturalistic perspective that steers clear of miraculous doctrines such as rebirth.

Spiritual Naturalist Society, spiritualnaturalistsociety.org

The Spiritual Naturalist Society encourages a naturalistic approach to practices often seen as spiritual, including but not limited to meditation.

Unitarian Universalist Buddhist Fellowship, http://uubf.org

The fellowship consists of practice groups affiliated with Unitarian Universalist congregations. Many have a secular orientation.

Glossary

compassion: A warm, positive feeling intended to alleviate suffering; not a sorrowful feeling.

empathy: Feeling what another person feels. This is not necessarily a positive feeling, because when one empathizes with the suffering of others, one suffers too.

meditation: Typically, practicing mindfulness with a narrow focus on one particular sensation, such as the breathing, hearing ambient sounds, or the feeling in one's feet while walking.

metta: Loving-kindness; an attitude that is friendly, kindly, or loving.

mindfulness: Paying attention to what is going on in the present moment with an attitude of *metta*.

non-self: The philosophical view that what we refer to as our "self" is an unfolding process rather than a permanent entity (e.g., a soul).

neuroplasticity: Changes to the brain that occur following a thought or action that may facilitate similar thoughts or actions in the future.

tonglen: A meditative practice of mentally taking in suffering and giving out compassion.

Endnotes

1   "Can 'Mindful' Meditation Increase Profits?" *BBC News*, January 29, 2013, www.bbc.com/news/business-21244171; Jan Hoffman, "How Meditation Might Boost Your Test Scores," *New York Times*, April 3, 2013, well.blogs.nytimes .com/2013/04/03/how-meditation-might-boost-your-test-scores/; Erik E. Solberg, Kurt-Arne Berglund, Oyvind Engen, Oivind Ekeberg, and Mitch Loeb, "The Effect of Meditation on Shooting Performance," *British Journal of Sports Medicine* 30, no. 4 (1996): 342–46; Mark Westmoquette, "Mindfulness for Rifle Shooters," *Outer Universe to Inner Universe* (blog), April 19, 2014, outerinner universe.blogspot.com/2014/04/mindfulness-for-rifle-shooters.html.

2   Kitty Dumas, "UM Researcher Helping Soldiers Battle Stress," *Miami Herald*, August 19, 2013, www.miamiherald.com/2013/08/19/3572882/um-researcher -helping-soldiers.html#storylink=cpy; Anna North, "The Mindfulness Backlash," *New York Times*, June 30, 2014, op-talk.blogs.nytimes.com/2014/06/30 /the-mindfulness-backlash/.

3   The exception to this may be people diagnosable as psychopaths. With physical alterations to the brain that apparently prevent them from feeling empathy, it may be difficult or impossible for psychopaths to cultivate compassion toward others.

4   Sharon Salzberg, *Lovingkindness: The Revolutionary Art of Happiness* (Boston: Shambhala, 1995), 57.

5   Acharya Buddharakkhita, *Metta: The Philosophy and Practice of Universal Love*, accessed March 16, 2014, www.accesstoinsight.org/lib/authors/buddharakkhita /wheel365.html.

6   Buddhaghosa, *The Path of Purification*, trans. Bhikkhu Ñāṇamoli (Kandy, Sri Lanka: Buddhist Publication Society, 2010), 292.

7   Ibid., 293.

8   Robert D. Putnam, "E Pluribus Unum: Diversity and Community in the

Twenty-First Century: The 2006 Johan Skytte Prize Lecture," *Scandinavian Political Studies* 30, no. 2 (2007): 137–74. One could reasonably suggest that increasing distrust is rational. But Putnam found that even among communities with the same crime rates, the more diverse communities had lower levels of trust. In highly diverse communities, people are less trusting even of members of their own ethnic group: it seems that people become more constricted in general. While this distrust may be driven by fear of people who are different, it is not necessarily founded on an accurate perception of risk.

9   *Millennials in Adulthood: Detached from Institutions, Networked with Friends,* Pew Research Center, March 7, 2014, www.pewsocialtrends.org/2014/03/07/millennials-in-adulthood/; Connie Cass, "Poll Reveals Americans Don't Trust Each Other Anymore," November 30, 2013, www.huffingtonpost.com/2013/11/30/poll-americans-trust_n_4363884.html.

10   "FAQs," Project Implicit, implicit.harvard.edu/implicit/demo/background/faqs.html#faq7, accessed June 25, 2013; Yoona Kang, Jeremy R. Gray, and John F. Dovidio, "The Nondiscriminating Heart: Lovingkindness Meditation Training Decreases Implicit Intergroup Bias," *Journal of Experimental Psychology: General* 143, no. 3 (June 2014): 1306–13.

11   Joe Keohane, "I, Causticus," *Boston,* July 2006.

12   Daphna McKnight, "Tonglen Meditation's Effect on Levels of Compassion and Self-Compassion: A Proof of Concept Study and Instructional Guide," thesis completed as part of the Upaya Buddhist Chaplaincy Training Program, 2010–12, upaya.org/uploads/pdfs/McKnightTonglenThesis.pdf.

13   Tania Singer and Matthias Bolz, eds., *Compassion: Bridging Practice and Science* (Munich: Max Planck Society, 2013), 275. E-book available at www.compassion-training.org/?page=download&lang=en.

14   "A Single Death Is a Tragedy; A Million Deaths Is a Statistic," Quote Investigator, May 21, 2010, quoteinvestigator.com/2010/05/21/death-statistic/.

15   Paul Slovic, "Numbed by Numbers," *Foreign Policy,* March 13, 2007, www.foreignpolicy.com/articles/2007/03/12/numbed_by_numbers; Deborah A. Small, George Loewenstein, and Paul Slovic, "Sympathy and Callousness: The Impact of Deliberative Thought on Donations to Identifiable and Statistical Victims," *Organizational Behavior and Human Decision Processes* 102, no. 2 (2007): 143–53; Paul Slovic, "If I Look at the Mass I Will Never Act: Psychic Numbing and Genocide," *Judgment and Decision Making* 2, no. 2 (2007): 79–95.

16   Kristin D. Neff, "Self-Compassion, Self-Esteem, and Well-Being," *Social and Personality Psychology Compass* 5, no. 1 (2011): 1–12; Kristin Neff, "Why We Should Stop Chasing Self-Esteem and Start Developing Self-Compassion," *Huffington Post,* April 6, 2011, www.huffingtonpost.com/kristin-neff/self-compassion_b_843721.html.

17   Jean M. Twenge, Sara Konrath, Joshua D. Foster, W. Keith Campbell, and Brad J. Bushman, "Egos Inflating over Time: A Cross-Temporal Meta-analysis of the Narcissistic Personality Inventory," *Journal of Personality* 76, no. 4 (2008): 875–902; Roy F. Baumeister, Brad J. Bushman, and W. Keith Campbell, "Self-Esteem,

Narcissism, and Aggression: Does Violence Result from Low Self-Esteem or from Threatened Egotism?" *Current Directions in Psychological Science* 9, no. 1 (2000): 26–29.

18   Kristin Neff, *Self-Compassion: Stop Beating Yourself Up and Leave Insecurity Behind* (New York: HarperCollins, 2011), 153.

19   David D. Burns, *Feeling Good: The New Mood Therapy* (New York: Morrow, 1980), 32–43.

20   Nirbhay N. Singh, Giulio E. Lancioni, Robert G. Wahler, Alan S. W. Winton, and Judy Singh, "Mindfulness Approaches in Cognitive Behavior Therapy," *Behavioural and Cognitive Psychotherapy* 36, no. 6 (2008): 659.

21   Carsten K. W. De Dreu, Lindred L. Greer, Gerben A. Van Kleef, Shaul Shalvi, and Michel J. J. Handgraaf, "Oxytocin Promotes Human Ethnocentrism," *Proceedings of the National Academy of Sciences* 108, no. 4 (2011): 1262–66; Carsten K. W. De Dreu, Lindred L. Greer, Michel J. J. Handgraaf, Shaul Shalvi, Gerben A. Van Kleef, Matthijs Baas, Femke S. Ten Velden, Eric Van Dijk, and Sander W. W. Feith, "The Neuropeptide Oxytocin Regulates Parochial Altruism in Intergroup Conflict among Humans," *Science* 328, no. 5984 (2010): 1408–11.

22   Anthony G. Greenwald and Thomas F. Pettigrew, "With Malice toward None and Charity for Some: Ingroup Favoritism Enables Discrimination," *American Psychologist* 69, no. 7 (October 2014): 669–84.

23   Andreas Bartels and Semir Zeki, "The Neural Correlates of Maternal and Romantic Love," *Neuroimage* 21, no. 3 (2004): 1155–66; Peter Kirsch, Christine Esslinger, Qiang Chen, Daniela Mier, Stefanie Lis, Sarina Siddhanti, Harald Gruppe, Venkata S. Mattay, Bernd Gallhofer, and Andreas Meyer-Lindenberg, "Oxytocin Modulates Neural Circuitry for Social Cognition and Fear in Humans," *Journal of Neuroscience* 25, no. 49 (2005): 11489–93; Matthias Gamer, Bartosz Zurowski, and Christian Büchel, "Different Amygdala Subregions Mediate Valence-Related and Attentional Effects of Oxytocin in Humans," *Proceedings of the National Academy of Sciences* 107, no. 20 (2010): 9400–9405; Moïra Mikolajczak, Nicolas Pinon, Anthony Lane, Philippe de Timary, and Olivier Luminet, "Oxytocin Not Only Increases Trust When Money Is at Stake, but Also When Confidential Information Is in the Balance," *Biological Psychology* 85, no. 1 (2010): 182–84.

24   Ashley Smith and Stacy Mattingly, *Unlikely Angel: The Untold Story of the Atlanta Hostage Hero* (Grand Rapids, MI: Zondervan, 2005).

25   V. L. Kettering, J. A. Barraza, P. Williams, M. L. Ly, C. Holcomb, C. A. Wolf, P. J. Zak, and M. L. Spezio, "Unique Effects of Metta Meditation on Eusocial Behavior," unpublished manuscript.

26   Paul J. Zak, *The Moral Molecule: The Source of Love and Prosperity* (New York: Dutton, 2012), 104.

27   Gregor Domes, Markus Heinrichs, Andre Michel, Christoph Berger, and Sabine C. Herpertz, "Oxytocin Improves 'Mind-Reading' in Humans," *Biological Psychiatry* 61, no. 6 (2007): 731–33.

28   Moïra Mikolajczak, James J. Gross, Anthony Lane, Olivier Corneille, Philippe

de Timary, and Olivier Luminet, "Oxytocin Makes People Trusting, Not Gullible," *Psychological Science* 21, no. 8 (2010): 1072–74.

29   Robert D. Hare, *Without Conscience: The Disturbing World of the Psychopaths among Us* (New York: Guilford Press, 1999), 74.

30   Ibid., 42–43.

31   Joseph Stromberg, "The Neuroscientist Who Discovered He Was a Psychopath," *Salon*, November 23, 2013, www.salon.com/2013/11/23/this_neuro scientist_discovered_he_was_a_psychopath_partner/.

32   Nikhil Swaminathan, "Why Does the Brain Need So Much Power?" *Scientific American*, April 29, 2008, www.scientificamerican.com/article/why-does-the -brain-need-s/.

33   Barbara L. Fredrickson, Michael A. Cohn, Kimberly A. Coffey, Jolynn Pek, and Sandra M. Finkel, "Open Hearts Build Lives: Positive Emotions, Induced through Loving-Kindness Meditation, Build Consequential Personal Resources," *Journal of Personality and Social Psychology* 95, no. 5 (2008): 1045; Michael A. Cohn and Barbara L. Fredrickson, "In Search of Durable Positive Psychology Interventions: Predictors and Consequences of Long-Term Positive Behavior Change," *Journal of Positive Psychology* 5, no. 5 (2010): 355–66.

34   C. Sue Carter, A. Courtney Devries, and Lowell L. Getz, "Physiological Substrates of Mammalian Monogamy: the Prairie Vole Model," *Neuroscience and Biobehavioral Reviews* 19, no. 2 (1995): 303–14.

35   Jennifer N. Ferguson, J. Matthew Aldag, Thomas R. Insel, and Larry J. Young, "Oxytocin in the Medial Amygdala is Essential for Social Recognition in the Mouse," *Journal of Neuroscience* 21, no. 20 (2001): 8278–85.

36   Zak, *Moral Molecule*, 61.

37   Jean Decety and Julie Grèzes, "The Power of Simulation: Imagining One's Own and Other's Behavior," *Brain Research* 1079, no. 1 (2006): 4–14; Ingo G. Meister, Timo Krings, Henrik Foltys, Babak Boroojerdi, M. Müller, R. Töpper, and A. Thron, "Playing Piano in the Mind: An fMRI Study on Music Imagery and Performance in Pianists," *Cognitive Brain Research* 19, no. 3 (2004): 219–28; Stephanie D. Preston and Frans de Waal, "Empathy: Its Ultimate and Proximate Bases," *Behavioral and Brain Sciences* 25, no. 1 (2002): 2.

38   Kjell Fuxe, Dasiel O. Borroto-Escuela, Wilber Romero-Fernandez, Francisco Ciruela, Paul Manger, Guiseppina Leo, Zaida Díaz-Cabiale, and Luigi F. Agnati, "On the Role of Volume Transmission and Receptor–Receptor Interactions in Social Behaviour: Focus on Central Catecholamine and Oxytocin Neurons," *Brain Research* 1476 (2012): 119–31; Wim B. J. Mens, Albert Witter, and Tjeerd B. Van Wimersma Greidanus, "Penetration of Neurohypophyseal Hormones from Plasma into Cerebrospinal Fluid (CSF): Half-Times of Disappearance of These Neuropeptides from CSF," *Brain Research* 262, no. 1 (1983): 143–49.

39   Ginger A. Hoffman, Anne Harrington, and Howard L. Fields, "Pain and the Placebo: What We Have Learned," *Perspectives in Biology and Medicine* 48, no. 2 (2005): 248–65; Jon D. Levine, Newton C. Gordon, and Howard L. Fields, "The Mechanism of Placebo Analgesia," *Lancet* 312, no. 8091 (1978): 654–57; Rick

Heller, "Buddhism's Pain Relief," *Buddhadharma* (Fall 2010): 34–41; Rick Heller, "Faith Healing for Skeptics: How the Expectant Brain Relieves Pain," *Tikkun*, November 10, 2011, www.tikkun.org/nextgen/faith-healing-for-skeptics-how-the-expectant-brain-relieves-pain.

40   Larry Rosenberg and David Guy, *Breath by Breath: The Liberating Practice of Insight Liberation* (Boston: Shambhala, 1998), 166.

41   The story is retold in Jack Kornfield, *Meditation for Beginners: Six Guided Meditations for Insight, Inner Clarity, and Cultivating a Compassionate Heart* (Boulder, CO: Sounds True, 2004), 35.

42   "Pain without Suffering: An Interview with Jon Kabat-Zinn," *Tricycle*, Winter 2002, www.tricycle.com/onpractice/pain-without-suffering.

43   Alvaro Pascual-Leone and Fernando Torres, "Plasticity of the Sensorimotor Cortex Representation of the Reading Finger in Braille Readers," *Brain* 116, no. 1 (1993): 39–52.

44   James Joyce, "A Painful Case," *Dubliners* (1914), www.online-literature.com/james_joyce/964/.

45   Edmund Jacobson, *Progressive Relaxation*, 2nd ed. (Chicago: University of Chicago Press, 1938), 309–13.

46   Anna Wise, *Awakening the Mind: A Guide to Harnessing the Power of Your Brainwaves* (Los Angeles: J. P. Tarcher, 2002), 36, emphasis in original.

47   Edmund Jacobson, *You Must Relax*, 5th ed. (New York: McGraw-Hill, 1978), 246.

48   This neuromuscular connection between thought, emotion, and muscular action has been shown in healthy adults. However, it appears that patients with paralysis can still experience the full repertoire of thoughts and emotions. See Femke Nijboer, S. P. Carmien, Enrique Leon, Fabrice O. Morin, Randal A. Koene, and Ulrich Hoffmann, "Affective Brain-Computer Interfaces: Psychophysiological Markers of Emotion in Healthy Persons and in Persons with Amyotrophic Lateral Sclerosis," *3rd International Conference on Affective Computing and Intelligent Interaction and Workshops* (Amsterdam: IEEE, 2009), 1–11. Apparently, muscular relaxation sends a feedback signal to the brain that can influence brain activity, but in the absence of any connectivity with the muscles, feedback doesn't enter into the equation.

49   On subvocalization, see F. J. McGuigan and Andrew B. Dollins, "Patterns of Covert Speech Behavior and Phonetic Coding," *Pavlovian Journal of Biological Science* 24, no. 1 (1989): 19–26; F. J. McGuigan and C. L. Winstead, "Discriminative Relationship between Covert Oral Behavior and the Phonemic System in Internal Information Processing," *Journal of Experimental Psychology* 103, no. 5 (1974): 885; Frank J. McGuigan, *Psychophysiological Measurement of Covert Behavior: A Guide for the Laboratory* (Hillsdale, NJ: L. Erlbaum Associates, 1979). On recognition of subvocal speech, see "Who's Who at NASA: Chuck Jorgensen," May 2004, www.nasatech.com/NEWS/May04/who_0504.html; Chuck Jorgensen and Kim Binsted, "Web Browser Control Using EMG Based Sub Vocal Speech Recognition," in *Proceedings of the 38th Annual Hawaii*

International Conference on System Sciences (Waikoloa Village, Hawaii, IEEE, 2005), 294c; Lisa Katayama, "Invention Awards: A Real-Life Babel Fish for the Speaking Impaired," *Popular Science*, May 20, 2009, www.popsci.com/scitech/article/2009-05/electronic-voice-box.

50   Paul M. Lehrer, "Progressive Relaxation," in *Principles and Practice of Stress Management*, ed. Paul M. Lehrer, Robert L. Woolfolk, and Wesley E. Sime (New York: Guilford, 2007), 57.

51   "Vitakkasanthana Sutta: The Relaxation of Thoughts," *Majjhima Nikaya: The Middle-Length Discourses*, trans. Thanissaro Bhikkhu (1997), www.accessto insight.org/tipitaka/mn/mn.020.than.html; according to the most relevant study I've found on immobilizing the tongue: "When children are asked to write with the mouth open or the tongue held between the teeth, writing errors greatly increase," apparently because these practices interfere with the generation of inner speech, which children in particular rely on to sound out words. See M. Perrone-Bertolotti, L. Rapin, J.-P. Lachaux, M. Baciu, and Hélène Loevenbruck, "What Is That Little Voice Inside My Head? Inner Speech Phenomenology, Its Role in Cognitive Performance, and Its Relation to Self-Monitoring," *Behavioural Brain Research* 261 (2014): 229, referencing Aleksandr Romanovich Luria, *Higher Cortical Functions in Man* (New York: Basic Books, 1966).

52   Pamela K. Adelmann and Robert B. Zajonc, "Facial Efference and the Experience of Emotion," *Annual Review of Psychology* 40, no. 1 (1989): 249–80; Andreas Hennenlotter, Christian Dresel, Florian Castrop, Andres O. Ceballos-Baumann, Afra M. Wohlschläger, and Bernhard Haslinger, "The Link between Facial Feedback and Neural Activity within Central Circuitries of Emotion: New Insights from Botulinum Toxin–Induced Denervation of Frown Muscles," *Cerebral Cortex* 19, no. 3 (2009): 537–42; David A. Havas, Arthur M. Glenberg, Karol A. Gutowski, Mark J. Lucarelli, and Richard J. Davidson, "Cosmetic Use of Botulinum Toxin-A Affects Processing of Emotional Language," *Psychological Science* 21 (July 2010): 895–900.

53   Charles Darwin, *The Expression of the Emotions in Man and Animals* (New York: Oxford University Press, 1998), 234, 359–60.

54   Alfons Schnitzler, Joachim Gross, and Lars Timmermann, "Synchronised Oscillations of the Human Sensorimotor Cortex," *Acta Neurobiologiae Experimentalis* 60, no. 2 (2000): 271–88; Alfons Schnitzler and Joachim Gross, "Normal and Pathological Oscillatory Communication in the Brain," *Nature Reviews Neuroscience* 6, no. 4 (2005): 285–96.

55   Joshua Ian Davis, Ann Senghas, and Kevin N. Ochsner, "How Does Facial Feedback Modulate Emotional Experience?" *Journal of Research in Personality* 43, no. 5 (2009): 822–29. Although lack of facial movement in healthy adults seems to dampen emotions, a woman with facial paralysis reported feeling normal levels of emotions. See Jocelyn M. Keillor, Anna M. Barrett, Gregory P. Crucian, Sarah Kortenkamp, and Kenneth M. Heilman, "Emotional Experience and Perception in the Absence of Facial Feedback," *Journal of the International Neuropsychological Society* 8, no. 1 (2002): 130–35.

56   Lehrer, "Progressive Relaxation," 57.

57   Herbert Benson, talk at Harvard Book Store, Cambridge, MA, July 13, 2010.

58   States News Service, "Meditating to Try to Lower Crime Rate," *New York Times*, August 1, 1993, www.nytimes.com/1993/08/01/nyregion/meditating -to-try-to-lower-crime-rate.html.

59   Manoj K. Bhasin, Jeffery A. Dusek, Bei-Hung Chang, Marie G. Joseph, John W. Denninger, Gregory L. Fricchione, Herbert Benson, and Towia A. Liber- mann, "Relaxation Response Induces Temporal Transcriptome Changes in En- ergy Metabolism, Insulin Secretion and Inflammatory Pathways," *PLOS One* 8, no. 5 (2013): e62817.

60   James H. Austin, *Meditating Selflessly: Practical Neural Zen* (Cambridge, MA: MIT Press, 2011), 67–68.

61   M. D. Hunter, S. B. Eickhoff, T. W. R. Miller, T. F. D. Farrow, I. D. Wilkinson, and P. W. R. Woodruff, "Neural Activity in Speech-Sensitive Auditory Cortex during Silence," *Proceedings of the National Academy of Sciences* 103, no. 1 (2006): 189–94.

62   The only problem with this bottom-up hypothesis is that it relies on studies that are thirty years old or more. Neuroscientists I've corresponded with were unable to point me toward any relevant studies that use recent brain-imaging techniques. This would be a hypothesis worthy of investigation with modern methods.

63   Bridget Murray Law, "Probing the Depression-Rumination Cycle: Why Chew- ing on Problems Just Makes Them Harder to Swallow," *Monitor on Psychology* 36, no. 10 (2005): 38–39.

64   Adapted from Paul Reps and Nyogen Senzaki, *Zen Flesh, Zen Bones: A Collection of Zen and Pre-Zen Writings* (Boston: Tuttle, 1985), 38–39.

65   Alan Baddeley, "Working Memory," *Science* 255, no. 5044 (1992): 556–59; Eraldo Paulesu, Christopher D. Frith, and Richard S. J. Frackowiak, "The Neural Cor- relates of the Verbal Component of Working Memory," *Nature* 362, no. 6418 (1993): 342–45.

66   Alan Baddeley, "Working Memory," *Current Biology* 20, no. 4 (2010): R136– R140; Giuseppe Vallar, Anna Maria Di Betta, and Maria Caterina Silveri, "The Phonological Short-Term Store-Rehearsal System: Patterns of Impairment and Neural Correlates," *Neuropsychologia* 35, no. 6 (1997): 795–812.

67   Jeff Martin, "The Otto Show," *The Simpsons*, season 3, episode 22, Fox, 1992, www.simpsonsarchive.com/episodes/8F21.html.

68   Colin A. Espie and Simon D. Kyle, "Primary Insomnia: An Overview of Practi- cal Management Using Cognitive Behavioral Techniques," *Sleep Medicine Clinics* 4, no. 4 (2009): 559–69.

69   Lehrer has studied mantra meditation. See Paul M. Lehrer, Robert L. Woolfolk, Anthony J. Rooney, Barbara McCann, and Patricia Carrington, "Progressive Relaxation and Meditation: A Study of Psychophysiological and Therapeutic Differences between Two Techniques," *Behaviour Research and Therapy* 21, no. 6 (1983): 651–62.

70   Matthew A. Killingsworth and Daniel T. Gilbert, "A Wandering Mind Is an Unhappy Mind," *Science* 330, no. 6006 (2010): 932.

71   Todd S. Braver and Jonathan D. Cohen, "On the Control of Control: The Role of Dopamine in Regulating Prefrontal Function and Working Memory," in Stephen Monsell and Jon Driver, *Control of Cognitive Processes* (Cambridge, MA: MIT Press, 2000).

72   William James, *Talks to Teachers on Psychology and to Students on Some of Life's Ideals* (Cambridge, MA: Harvard University Press, 1983), 68.

73   Mihaly Csikszentmihalyi, *Flow: The Psychology of Optimal Experience* (New York: Harper & Row, 1990), 107.

74   David Shenk, *The Forgetting: Alzheimer's, Portrait of an Epidemic* (New York: Doubleday, 2001), 193.

75   Robert D. Hare, *Without Conscience: The Disturbing World of the Psychopaths among Us* (New York: Guilford Press, 1999), 88.

76   Rick Heller, "Buddhism's Pain Relief," *Buddhadharma* (Fall 2010): 34–41.

77   For a discussion of the origin of the Serenity Prayer, see Elisabeth Sifton, *The Serenity Prayer: Faith and Politics in Times of Peace and War* (New York: Norton, 2003), 277. Niebuhr cites Epictetus in Reinhold Niebuhr, *The Nature and Destiny of Man* (New York: Charles Scribner's Sons, 1941), 291. The quote from Epictetus is in *Arrian's Discourses of Epictetus*, in *The Stoic and Epicurean Philosophers*, ed. Whitney J. Oates (New York: Modern Library, 1940), 225.

78   Wendell Piez, "The Rain of Law," *Tricycle*, Winter 1992, www.tricycle.com /ancestors/the-rain-law; the term *mindfulness* was first used as a translation of the Pali word *sati* in 1881 by the British scholar Thomas W. Rhys Davids. See Robert E. Buswell Jr. and Donald S. Lopez Jr., "Which Mindfulness? The Modern Understanding of Mindfulness Differs Significantly from What the Term Has Historically Meant in Buddhism," *Tricycle*, May 8, 2014, www.tricycle.com /blog/which-mindfulness.

79   Henry David Thoreau, *Walden*, in *Walden and Other Writings* (New York: Bantam, 1981), 117.

80   Ibid., 188.

81   Ibid., 202–3.

82   Henry David Thoreau, *A Week on the Concord and Merrimack Rivers*, in *Walden and Other Writings* (New York: Bantam, 1981), 65–66.

83   Ralph Waldo Emerson, "Nature," in *Selected Essays* (New York: Penguin, 1982), 38.

84   Marcus Aurelius, *Meditations*, trans. Maxwell Staniforth (New York: Penguin, 1964), 59.

85   Epictetus, *The Manual of Epictetus*, in *The Stoic and Epicurean Philosophers* (New York: Modern Library, 1940), 489.

86   Marcus Aurelius, *Meditations*, 98.

87   Thomas McEvilley, *The Shape of Ancient Thought: Comparative Studies in Greek and Indian Philosophies* (New York: Allworth, 2002), 14; Stephen Batchelor, *Confession of a Buddhist Atheist* (New York: Spiegel & Grau, 2010), 248.

88   Apsley Cherry-Garrard, *The Worst Journey in the World* (New York: Carroll & Graf, 1989), 42. The first definition in a Google search for *stoic* is "a person who can endure pain or hardship without showing their feelings or complaining."

89   Johann Wolfgang von Goethe, *Italian Journey*, trans. W. H. Auden and Elizabeth Mayer (London: Penguin, 1970), 197.

90   Tony Hiss, *In Motion: The Experience of Travel* (New York: Alfred A. Knopf, 2010), 3.

91   Oliver R. W. Pergams and Patricia A. Zaradic, "Is Love of Nature in the US Becoming Love of Electronic Media? 16-Year Downtrend in National Park Visits Explained by Watching Movies, Playing Video Games, Internet Use, and Oil Prices," *Journal of Environmental Management* 80, no. 4 (2006): 387–93.

92   U Silananda, *The Four Foundations of Mindfulness* (Boston: Wisdom, 1990), 57.

93   Susan R. Barry, *Fixing My Gaze: A Scientist's Journey into Seeing in Three Dimensions* (New York: Basic Books, 2009), xii–xiii.

94   On loss of depth perception while under stress, see Dave Grossman and Loren W. Christensen, *On Combat: The Psychology and Physiology of Deadly Conflict in War and in Peace*, 3rd ed. (Millstadt, IL: Warrior Science, 2008), 47. On the evolution of depth perception, see Robert A. Barton, "Binocularity and Brain Evolution in Primates," *Proceedings of the National Academy of Sciences* 101, no. 27 (2004): 10113–15; Matt Cartmill, "Rethinking Primate Origins," *Science* 184, no. 4135 (1974): 436–43; Rick Hanson, "Just One Thing: Pet the Lizard," *Greater Good*, July 20, 2011, greatergood.berkeley.edu/article/item/just_one_thing _pet_the_lizard. I have twice attended workshops by Rick Hanson at the Barre Center for Buddhist Studies in which he discussed meditation from the perspective of neuroscience. Much of this information can be found in Rick Hanson and Richard Mendius, *Buddha's Brain: The Practical Neuroscience of Happiness, Love, and Wisdom* (Oakland, CA: New Harbinger, 2009).

95   Michael A. Cohen and Stephen Grossberg, "Neural Dynamics of Brightness Perception: Features, Boundaries, Diffusion, and Resonance," *Perception and Psychophysics* 36, no. 5 (1984): 428–56.

96   Dalai Lama, *Beyond Religion: Ethics for a Whole World* (Boston: Houghton Mifflin Harcourt, 2011), 166.

97   Fehmi is a psychologist who specializes in brain-wave biofeedback, a method by which subjects use real-time information from devices that measure brain waves in order to train their brains to achieve desired states. The efficacy of this method has been questioned, but the American Psychological Association website suggests it may be effective for treatment of attention deficit–hyperactivity disorder. See also Julia Anna Glombiewski, Kathrin Bernardy, and Winfried Häuser, "Efficacy of EMG- and EEG-Biofeedback in Fibromyalgia Syndrome: A Meta-analysis and a Systematic Review of Randomized Controlled Trials," *Evidence-Based Complementary and Alternative Medicine 2013*, no. 1 (2013): 1–11; American Psychological Association, "Getting in Touch with Your Inner Brainwaves through Biofeedback," November 10, 2003, www.apa.org/research/action /biofeedback.aspx.

98   Rachel Carson and Charles Pratt, *The Sense of Wonder* (New York: Harper & Row, 1965), 67.

99   Minkyung Koo, Sara B. Algoe, Timothy D. Wilson, and Daniel T. Gilbert, "It's a Wonderful Life: Mentally Subtracting Positive Events Improves People's Affective States, Contrary to Their Affective Forecasts," *Journal of Personality and Social Psychology* 95, no. 5 (2008): 1217–24.

100   Linda A. Henkel, "Point-and-Shoot Memories: The Influence of Taking Photos on Memory for a Museum Tour," *Psychological Science* 25, no. 2 (2014): 396–402.

101   Betty Edwards, *Drawing on the Right Side of the Brain* (Los Angeles: J. P. Tarcher, 1979), 52.

102   Viktor Shklovsky, "Art as Technique," in *Russian Formalist Criticism: Four Essays*, ed. Lee T. Lemon and Marion J. Reis (Lincoln: University of Nebraska Press, 1965), 13.

103   Thich Nhat Hanh and Lilian Cheung, *Savor: Mindful Eating, Mindful Life* (New York: HarperCollins: 2010), 126–27; Pam Belluck, "Obesity Rates Hit Plateau in U.S., Data Suggest," *New York Times*, January 13, 2010, www.nytimes.com /2010/01/14/health/14obese.html; Jaime Holguin, "Fast Food Linked to Child Obesity," January 5, 2004, Associated Press, www.cbsnews.com /stories/2004/01/05/health/main591325.shtml; Corby K. Martin, Stephen D. Anton, Heather Walden, Cheryl Arnett, Frank L. Greenway, and Donald A. Williamson, "Slower Eating Rate Reduces the Food Intake of Men, but Not Women: Implications for Behavioral Weight Control," *Behaviour Research and Therapy* 45, no. 10 (2007): 2349; M. Shah, J. Copeland, L. Dart, B. Adams-Huet, A. James, and D. Rhea, "Slower Eating Speed Lowers Energy Intake in Normal-Weight but Not Overweight/Obese Subjects," *Journal of the Academy of Nutrition and Dietetics* 114, no. 3 (2014): 393.

104   "Heartbreak and Ice Cream," *TV Tropes*, http://tvtropes.org/pmwiki/pmwiki .php/Main/HeartbreakAndIceCream, accessed April 3, 2015.

105   Barbara Ehrenreich, *Bright-Sided: How the Relentless Promotion of Positive Thinking Has Undermined America* (Waterville, ME: Thorndike, 2010), 284–96.

106   Daniel Kahneman and Angus Deaton, "High Income Improves Evaluation of Life but Not Emotional Well-Being," *Proceedings of the National Academy of Sciences* 107, no. 38 (2010): 16489–93.

107   Roy F. Baumeister, Kathleen D. Vohs, Jennifer L. Aaker, and Emily N. Garbinsky, "Some Key Differences between a Happy Life and a Meaningful Life," *Journal of Positive Psychology* 8, no. 6 (2013): 505–16.

108   Daniel J. Siegel, *The Mindful Brain: Reflection and Attunement in the Cultivation of Well-Being* (New York: W. W. Norton, 2007), 105.

109   Richard Restak, *The Brain* (New York: Warner, 1979), 99.

110   Siegel, *The Mindful Brain*, 106.

111   Marc G. Berman, John Jonides, and Stephen Kaplan, "The Cognitive Benefits of Interacting with Nature," *Psychological Science* 19, no. 12 (2008): 1207–12; Rebecca A. Clay, "Green Is Good for You," *Monitor in Psychology* 32 (2001): 40.

112   Alexander J. Shackman, Tim V. Salomons, Heleen A. Slagter, Andrew S. Fox,

Jameel J. Winter, and Richard J. Davidson, "The Integration of Negative Affect, Pain and Cognitive Control in the Cingulate Cortex," *Nature Reviews Neuroscience* 12, no. 3 (2011): 154–67.

113   Daniel M. Wegner, "Ironic Processes of Mental Control," *Psychological Review* 101, no. 1 (1994): 34; Jason P. Mitchell, Todd F. Heatherton, William M. Kelley, Carrie L. Wyland, Daniel M. Wegner, and C. Neil Macrae, "Separating Sustained from Transient Aspects of Cognitive Control during Thought Suppression," *Psychological Science* 18, no. 4 (2007): 292–97.

114   Matthew D. Lieberman, Naomi I. Eisenberger, Molly J. Crockett, Sabrina M. Tom, Jennifer H. Pfeifer, and Baldwin M. Way, "Putting Feelings into Words: Affect Labeling Disrupts Amygdala Activity in Response to Affective Stimuli," *Psychological Science* 18, no. 5 (2007): 421–28.

115   Narayana Manjunatha, Christoday Raja Jayant Khess, and Dushad Ram, "The Conceptualization of Terms: 'Mood' and 'Affect' in Academic Trainees of Mental Health," *Indian Journal of Psychiatry* 51, no. 4 (2009): 285. On labeling emotions, see Elisha Goldstein, *The Now Effect: How a Mindful Moment Can Change the Rest of Your Life* (London: Simon & Schuster, 2013), 252.

116   J. David Creswell, Baldwin M. Way, Naomi I. Eisenberger, and Matthew D. Lieberman, "Neural Correlates of Dispositional Mindfulness during Affect Labeling," *Psychosomatic Medicine* 69, no. 6 (2007): 560–65.

117   Matthew D. Lieberman, Tristen K. Inagaki, Golnaz Tabibnia, and Molly J. Crockett, "Subjective Responses to Emotional Stimuli during Labeling, Reappraisal, and Distraction," *Emotion* 11, no. 3 (2011): 468–80.

118   Katharina Kircanski, Matthew D. Lieberman, and Michelle G. Craske, "Feelings into Words: Contributions of Language to Exposure Therapy," *Psychological Science* 23, no. 10 (2012): 1086–91; Doris E. Payer, Kate Baicy, Matthew D. Lieberman, and Edythe D. London, "Overlapping Neural Substrates between Intentional and Incidental Down-Regulation of Negative Emotions," *Emotion* 12, no. 2 (2012): 229–35.

119   Melanie Thernstrom, *The Pain Chronicles: Cures, Myths, Mysteries, Prayers, Diaries, Brain Scans, Healing, and the Science of Suffering* (New York: Farrar, Straus and Giroux, 2010), 259–60.

120   Bill DeMain, "Music History #3: "Yes! We Have No Bananas," Mental Floss, July 21, 2012, mentalfloss.com/article/31253/music-history-3-yes-we-have-no-bananas.

121   Daniel Nettle, *Happiness: The Science behind Your Smile* (New York: Oxford University Press, 2005), 31–32.

122   Tara Brach, *Radical Acceptance: Embracing Your Life with the Heart of a Buddha* (New York: Bantam, 2003), 81–82.

123   James Olds and Peter Milner, "Positive Reinforcement Produced by Electrical Stimulation of Septal Area and Other Regions of Rat Brain," *Journal of Comparative and Physiological Psychology* 47, no. 6 (1954): 419–27; Richard F. Thompson, "James Olds: 1922–1976," *American Journal of Psychology* 92 (1979): 151–52.

124   Kent C. Berridge, "Pleasures of the Brain," *Brain and Cognition* 52, no. 1 (2003):

106–28. On the ethical aspects of such studies, see Alan Baumeister, "The Tulane Electrical Brain Stimulation Program: A Historical Case Study in Medical Ethics," *Journal of the History of the Neurosciences* 9, no. 3 (2000): 262–78. It should also be noted that many Buddhists take exception to all animal research.

125   Kent C. Berridge and Elliot S. Valenstein, "What Psychological Process Mediates Feeding Evoked by Electrical Stimulation of the Lateral Hypothalamus?" *Behavioral Neuroscience* 105, no. 1 (1991): 3–14.

126   Rebecca L. McMillan, Scott Barry Kaufman, and Jerome L. Singer, "Ode to Positive Constructive Daydreaming," *Frontiers in Psychology* 4 (2013): 1–9.

127   Gil Fronsdal, "The Spectrum of Desire," August 25, 2006, www.insight meditationcenter.org/books-articles/articles/the-spectrum-of-desire/.

128   "Indianapolis 500 Pre-Race," ABC, May 24, 2009.

129   What's happening, I speculate, is that mindfulness and complex deliberative thought both use working memory, and at some point the system gets overloaded. The evidence that mindfulness improves working memory implies that mindfulness makes use of working memory. However, if working memory is being taxed by the complex demands of, say, figuring out a complex logical problem, adding an additional load to it by practicing mindfulness may result in overload and frustration. By analogy, weightlifting builds muscles, but placing extra weights on top of a crate that you are trying to move may not be helpful. On mindfulness and working memory, see, for instance, Fadel Zeidan, Susan K. Johnson, Bruce J. Diamond, Zhanna David, and Paula Goolkasian, "Mindfulness Meditation Improves Cognition: Evidence of Brief Mental Training," *Consciousness and Cognition* 19, no. 2 (2010): 597–605; Michael D. Mrazek, Michael S. Franklin, Dawa Tarchin Phillips, Benjamin Baird, and Jonathan W. Schooler, "Mindfulness Training Improves Working Memory Capacity and GRE Performance while Reducing Mind Wandering," *Psychological Science* (2013): 776–81.

130   "Magga-vibhanga Sutta: An Analysis of the Path," *Samyutta Nikaya: The Grouped Discourses*, trans. Thanissaro Bhikkhu (1996), available at Access to Insight, www.accesstoinsight.org/tipitaka/sn/sn45/sn45.008.than.html.

131   Roy F. Baumeister, Brad J. Bushman, and W. Keith Campbell, "Self-Esteem, Narcissism, and Aggression: Does Violence Result from Low Self-Esteem or from Threatened Egotism?" *Current Directions in Psychological Science* 9, no. 1 (2000): 26–29; Brendan Nyhan and Jason Reifler, "Opening the Political Mind? The Effects of Self-Affirmation and Graphical Information on Factual Misperceptions," unpublished manuscript (2011).

132   Marshall B. Rosenberg, *Nonviolent Communication: A Language of Life*, 2nd ed. (Encinitas, CA: PuddleDancer, 2003).

133   John L. Allen Jr., "Doctrinal Jousting: Theologian's Work Raises Ire of Vatican, as Well as Questions about Authority, Process and the Limits of Scholarship," *National Catholic Reporter*, February 25, 2005.

134   Henry David Thoreau, *A Week on the Concord and Merrimack Rivers*, in *Walden and Other Writings* (New York: Bantam, 1981), 64.

135   Huston Smith, *The World's Religions* (San Francisco: HarperSanFrancisco, 1991), 82.

136   Benjamin Franklin, *The Autobiography of Benjamin Franklin* (Cedar Lake, MI: ReadaClassic, 2010), 86.

137   Roy F. Baumeister and John Tierney, *Willpower: Rediscovering the Greatest Human Strength* (New York: Penguin, 2011), 48–51, 156–59.

138   Dave Grossman and Loren W. Christensen, *On Combat: The Psychology and Physiology of Deadly Conflict in War and in Peace*, 3rd ed. (Millstadt, IL: Warrior Science, 2008), 75.

139   Britta K. Hölzel, James Carmody, Mark Vangel, Christina Congleton, Sita M. Yerramsetti, Tim Gard, and Sara W. Lazar, "Mindfulness Practice Leads to Increases in Regional Brain Gray Matter Density," *Psychiatry Research: Neuroimaging* 191, no. 1 (2011): 36–43.

140   Peter M. Gollwitzer, Ute C. Bayer, and Kathleen C. McCulloch, "The Control of the Unwanted," *New Unconscious* (2005): 485–515.

141   Gregory S. Berns, Samuel M. McClure, Giuseppe Pagnoni, and P. Read Montague, "Predictability Modulates Human Brain Response to Reward," *Journal of Neuroscience* 21, no. 8 (2001): 2793–98; Wolfram Schultz, "Predictive Reward Signal of Dopamine Neurons," *Journal of Neurophysiology* 80, no. 1 (1998): 1–27; Hannah M. Bayer and Paul W. Glimcher, "Midbrain Dopamine Neurons Encode a Quantitative Reward Prediction Error Signal," *Neuron* 47, no. 1 (2005): 129–41.

142   Stephen Batchelor, *Confession of a Buddhist Atheist* (New York: Spiegel & Grau, 2010), 179.

143   William H. McNeill, *Plagues and Peoples* (Garden City, NY: Anchor Press/ Doubleday, 1976), 137–40.

144   On brain activity during meditation, see Wendy Hasenkamp, Christine D. Wilson-Mendenhall, Erica Duncan, and Lawrence W. Barsalou, "Mind Wandering and Attention during Focused Meditation: A Fine-Grained Temporal Analysis of Fluctuating Cognitive States," *Neuroimage* 59, no. 1 (2012): 750–60. On brain areas active during inner chatter, see M. D. Hunter, S. B. Eickhoff, T. W. R. Miller, T. F. D. Farrow, I. D. Wilkinson, and P. W. R. Woodruff, "Neural Activity in Speech-Sensitive Auditory Cortex during Silence," *Proceedings of the National Academy of Sciences* 103, no. 1 (2006): 189–94; Istvan Molnar-Szakacs and Lucina Q. Uddin, "Self-Processing and the Default Mode Network: Interactions with the Mirror Neuron System," *Frontiers in Human Neuroscience* 7 (2013): 88–98.

145   On mindfulness meditation and long-term changes to the brain, see Britta K. Hölzel, James Carmody, Mark Vangel, Christina Congleton, Sita M. Yerramsetti, Tim Gard, and Sara W. Lazar, "Mindfulness Practice Leads to Increases in Regional Brain Gray Matter Density," *Psychiatry Research: Neuroimaging* 191, no. 1 (2011): 36–43. On long-term meditators who do compassion meditation, see Antoine Lutz, Julie Brefczynski-Lewis, Tom Johnstone, and Richard J. Davidson, "Regulation of the Neural Circuitry of Emotion by Compassion Meditation: Effects of Meditative Expertise," *PLOS One* 3, no. 3 (2008): e1897.

146   Joseph Breuer and Sigmund Freud, *Studies on Hysteria* (New York: Basic Books, 2009), 305.

147   Antonio R. Damasio, *Descartes' Error* (New York: Grosset/Putnam, 1994), 34–51.
148   Charles Darwin, "Notes on Marriage," Darwin Correspondence Project, www.darwinproject.ac.uk/darwins-notes-on-marriage, accessed November 2, 2014.
149   Malcolm Gladwell, *Blink: The Power of Thinking without Thinking* (New York: Little, Brown, 2005), 6–8.
150   See Chris Mooney, *The Republican Brain: The Science of Why They Deny Science and Reality* (Hoboken, NJ: Wiley, 2012), 29–41 for a discussion of motivated reasoning. Although Mooney mostly beats up on Republicans in the book, he acknowledges that motivated reasoning is a universal human tendency.
151   Elliot L. Atlas, Kirby C. Donnelly, C. S. Giam, and Andrew R. McFarland, "Chemical and Biological Characterization of Emissions from a Fireperson Training Facility," *American Industrial Hygiene Association Journal* 46, no. 9 (1985): 532–40.
152   Madhav Goyal, Sonal Singh, Erica M. S. Sibinga, Neda F. Gould, Anastasia Rowland-Seymour, Ritu Sharma, Zackary Berger, et al., "Meditation Programs for Psychological Stress and Well-Being: A Systematic Review and Meta-analysis," *JAMA Internal Medicine* 174, no. 3 (2014): 357–68.
153   Mary Garden, "Can Meditation Be Bad for You?" *Humanist*, September–October 2007.
154   Caleb Daniloff, "Treating Tibet's Traumatized: SPH's Michael Grodin Blends Eastern Healing and Western Medicine to Aid Torture Victims," *Bostonia*, Fall 2009.
155   Willoughby Britton, "BG 232: The Dark Night Project," *Buddhist Geeks*, September 2011, www.buddhistgeeks.com/2011/09/bg-232-the-dark-night-project.
156   Herbert Benson, *The Relaxation Response* (New York: Morrow, 1975), 172.
157   Juliane Eberth and Peter Sedlmeier, "The Effects of Mindfulness Meditation: A Meta-analysis," *Mindfulness* 3, no. 3 (2012): 174–89; Bei-Hung Chang, Jeffery A. Dusek, and Herbert Benson, "Psychobiological Changes from Relaxation Response Elicitation: Long-Term Practitioners vs. Novices," *Psychosomatics* 52, no. 6 (2011): 550–59.
158   On cell aging, see Tonya L. Jacobs, Elissa S. Epel, Jue Lin, Elizabeth H. Blackburn, Owen M. Wolkowitz, David A. Bridwell, Anthony P. Zanesco, et al., "Intensive Meditation Training, Immune Cell Telomerase Activity, and Psychological Mediators," *Psychoneuroendocrinology* 36, no. 5 (2011): 664–81; Elissa Epel, Jennifer Daubenmier, Judith Tedlie Moskowitz, Susan Folkman, and Elizabeth Blackburn, "Can Meditation Slow Rate of Cellular Aging? Cognitive Stress, Mindfulness, and Telomeres," *Annals of the New York Academy of Sciences* 1172, no. 1 (2009): 34–53; on cortical thinning, see Sara W. Lazar, Catherine E. Kerr, Rachel H. Wasserman, Jeremy R. Gray, Douglas N. Greve, Michael T. Treadway, Metta McGarvey, et al., "Meditation Experience Is Associated with Increased Cortical Thickness," *Neuroreport* 16, no. 17 (2005): 1893.
159   Frieder R. Lang, David Weiss, Denis Gerstorf, and Gert G. Wagner,

"Forecasting Life Satisfaction across Adulthood: Benefits of Seeing a Dark Future?" *Psychology and Aging* 28, no. 1 (2013): 249. However, others have found that positive feelings can increase longevity. See, for instance, Ed Diener and Micaela Y. Chan, "Happy People Live Longer: Subjective Well-Being Contributes to Health and Longevity," *Applied Psychology: Health and Well-Being* 3, no. 1 (2011): 1–43. Mindfulness calls not for optimism but for a kindhearted realism. More research on these questions is needed.

160   Regarding World War II, see Brian Daizen Victoria, *Zen at War* (Lanham, MD: Rowman & Littlefield, 2006), 95–129; Dale S. Wright, "Satori and the Moral Dimension of Enlightenment," *Journal of Buddhist Ethics* 13 (2006): 1–17. Regarding contemporary violence, see Tim Hume, "Dalai Lama to Myanmar, Sri Lanka Buddhists: Stop Violence against Muslims," CNN, July 7, 2014, www.cnn.com/2014/07/07/world/asia/dalai-lama-muslim-violence/; regarding recent scandals, see Kevin Douglas Grant, "Sexual Abuse Allegations Give Pause to US Buddhist Community," *Global Post*, February 13, 2013, www.globalpost.com/dispatches/globalpost-blogs/belief/sexual-abuse-allegations-buddhist-community.

161   James H. Austin, *Zen and the Brain: Toward an Understanding of Meditation and Consciousness* (Cambridge, MA: MIT Press, 1998), 536–38.

162   Sam Harris, *Waking Up* (New York: Simon & Schuster, 2014), 81–119.

163   For a discussion of how non-self should be interpreted not as a metaphysical doctrine but rather as a mental strategy to reduce one's suffering, see Thanissaro Bhikkhu, "Selflessness: The Not-Self Strategy," 1993, enlight.lib.ntu.edu.tw/FULLTEXT/JR-AN/an142381.pdf.

164   Willoughby Britton, "BG 232: The Dark Night Project," *Buddhist Geeks*, September 2011, www.buddhistgeeks.com/2011/09/bg-232-the-dark-night-project.

165   Thanissaro Bhikkhu, *With Each and Every Breath: A Guide to Meditation* (Valley Center, CA: Metta Forest Monastery, 2012), 2–11.

Index

About the Author

FREELANCE JOURNALIST and meditation instructor Rick Heller has reported for the *Lowell Sun* and other New England newspapers and has been published in *Buddhadharma*, *UUWorld*, *Tikkun*, *Free Inquiry*, *Faith Street*, *The Humanist*, and *Boston* magazines. He has contributed short stories to *Fantasy and Science Fiction*.

Rick is the facilitator of the Humanist Mindfulness Group and has led meditations sponsored by the Humanist Community at Harvard since 2009. He has also attended workshops and retreats at the Cambridge Insight Meditation Center, the Barre Center for Buddhist Studies, and the Insight Meditation Society.

He holds a bachelor of science degree in electrical engineering from MIT, a master's degree in public policy from Harvard University, and a master of science degree in journalism from Boston University.

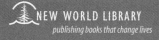